Upbeat

Growing resilience and positivity in the face of medical adversity

BETH GREENAWAY

RƎTHINK PRESS

First published in Great Britain 2018
by Rethink Press (www.rethinkpress.com)

Cover image © Shutterstock / Aksabir

Contents

Why I Wrote This Book

People may say that I have had more than my fair share of serious health challenges. If I look at the bare facts – three open-heart surgeries, a stroke which left me blind in my left eye, and, most recently, a serious infection in my heart that almost cost me my life – then I could be inclined to agree. But I don't.

The opposite is true, and those seemingly traumatic events have instead had a positive effect on my life and gone a long way to making me the person I am today. I have grown immeasurably as a result, and I honestly wouldn't change a thing.

As much as I nurture my positivity and have a strong mindset, though, some days are still a struggle. I have cried (a lot), felt angry, been resentful towards others whom I perceive have an easy life, got lost in self-pity, and even questioned the point in carrying on at all when it feels like everything is against me.

I wouldn't be truthful if I didn't confess that I experience fear and anxiety, get depressed, and sometimes just want to feel sorry for myself and get fully immersed in the 'why me?' experience. The only rule I have is not to allow myself to stay in that dark place for long. I know I'm worth more than that!

More than once I have had to face my own mortality, and every day I get regular reminders that I have been forever changed by what has happened. I couldn't undo the past even if I wanted to, but I can do my best to move towards my future with optimism. I refuse to be a victim of my circumstances, as in doing so I would surrender my self-esteem, hope and, ultimately, happiness.

I would describe myself as a realistic optimist. I recognise that life can be hard for everyone, but it is also the most incredible gift. I am grateful to have grown up in a loving family, to have supportive friends, to live in a country where I feel safe, and to be surrounded by the opportunity to be and do almost anything.

Over the years, probably thousands of complete strangers have played their part in keeping me alive – not just the obvious ones, but radiographers, admin staff, people who have donated blood, lab technicians, porters and countless others. If I think about that amount of compassion and care – even if I could actually believe that it was 'just doing their job' – then it is impossible not to feel grateful.

It would be easy to view my medical challenges as predominantly negative, but instead I recognise how much they have shaped and defined my character. I have built inner strength and resilience, which positively impacts many areas of my life. I feel gratitude and not resentment.

In my younger days, I saw myself as a victim and wore the badge for believing that life had dealt me a bad card. To transform my thinking has taken years of soul-searching and self-analysis, and, perhaps most importantly, the love and support of some key individuals.

I have often been perplexed by the idea that we bounce back from adversity, as that rather implies that the struggle is to be the same person we were before. If adversity teaches us anything, it is that we have the courage to survive, learn from the experience and become a better human being as a result. If we get it right, we bounce forward and not back!

Trauma of any sort often involves some form of loss, starting with that of our old identity. In a split second, our perceptions about ourselves, the fairness of life, and our hopes and expectations for the future can be irreparably altered. Bouncing 'back' and establishing a new normal require a lot of soul-searching and contemplation. Although the support of others can help, much of the work needs to be done alone. Establishing a new set of values and goals is unique to the individual, and it requires a higher level of self-awareness and determination.

It is human nature to crave stability and control – factors that can be lost when you face a long-term health condition. I have certainly found it hard to deal with the unpredictability of my illness and the way it can catch me off guard with fluctuating energy levels, unplanned hospitalisations and enforced modifications to my life plan. I have developed a nervous acceptance that the stability of my health can be shattered at any time, yet I choose not to live in fear of that event.

I have learned to pursue my dreams and to do my best to go confidently towards my future despite that uncertainty. I refuse to base my life decisions on an identity as a 'sick person', or to act as if there is a sword of Damocles hanging over my head. Nobody wants to be around a self-obsessed person or one who is locked in self-pity, so I have learned to put on a brave face to the world, even if at times it conceals the turmoil inside.

As well as dealing with modifying my own expectations of myself and my capabilities, I have had to accept that others do not walk in my shoes and cannot always be expected to understand how I feel. I would bet that anyone who lives with a long-term illness has had to deal with the perceptions of others, which can go from thinking we are miraculously cured to seeing us as irretrievably broken. Neither stance is helpful.

Introduction

If we are to thrive after adversity, we must accept where we are now and then come up with a realistic plan to bounce forward. It is not easy, and there are inescapable daily reminders of how we have been changed by our health challenges and the limitations that these impose. Hospital appointments, daily medication, symptoms and, for some, noticeable physical disabilities all single us out as being different.

We all feel inspired when we hear stories of triumph over unbelievable adversity. When we watch the Paralympics or the Invictus Games, we admire the ability of the competitors to keep striving to make the most of life. Yet all too often in the face of our own struggles, we conclude that those achievements are in some way reserved for people who are more remarkable than us.

I truly believe that we are all amazing in our own way. Far from being a negative, our journey and the way we deal with setbacks can be a springboard for remarkable personal growth. Rather than struggling to rebuild ourselves as we were before, there is an opportunity to bounce forward – stronger, wiser and more resilient. It just takes courage and a willingness to try.

Recovery from health adversity is an ongoing process, which is often punctuated by further challenges. The biggest key to healing my mind and body has been to stop focussing on myself and instead do my best to help others. That evolution has not been smooth or easy, but I have grown spiritually, emotionally and mentally as a result.

While looking at the important factors in my own recovery, I have sought to understand how we can increase our likelihood of growing from adversity. I have always been intrigued by why some individuals seem to evolve and thrive after a life-changing event, yet others get stuck and are unable to move beyond what has happened to them. People can get lost in a cycle of depression and anxiety, or even suffer from post-traumatic stress.

It is not all doom and gloom. Undoubtedly, some people who face significant adversity can experience very positive changes as a result. There is always a period of acceptance and adjustment, but that can give rise to a new perspective and personal growth. For those who need it, there is undoubtedly a place for formal counselling and intervention, but I am a big believer that we can also do much to help ourselves.

What character traits make us resilient, and are those skills inherent in us or can they be learned? Is there a recipe for growth after adversity, and is it possible to guide people through that process? As you have probably guessed from the fact that I have written this book, I strongly believe the answer is yes!

Over the years I have developed coping strategies, many of which have been assets but some of which have held me back. Only by deliberately taking the time to understand my deepest thoughts and beliefs, and, more importantly, why I feel that way, have I been able to identify which is which. There are lessons here that can be learned.

I have always been one to actively seek answers to my problems and ways to expand my knowledge. This has come by talking to experts, attending courses and, perhaps most of all, reading books. There are many books about improving mental health, overcoming depression, and coping with anxiety and stress, and there are tens of thousands about how to stay physically healthy. Yet few of them give specific advice about living with a long-term physical illness and the day-to-day challenges that this can present.

Medical innovation means that many more people are living longer with a life-changing health condition. Often, this is not one big event that we have to come to terms with, but an ongoing journey which is frequently punctuated by further difficulties and obstacles.

Much of my work over the last ten years has centred on helping people with long-term health conditions to improve their fitness. Observing how other people deal with difficult health situations has taught me a great deal about how to cope better with my own. It has been a real honour to share parts of that journey with my clients, and to recognise how much we all need each other. That shared experience and empathy is a powerful part of recovery.

I have also come to understand the prevalence of significant adversity in everyone's lives. There is no such thing as an easy life, and I am not even sure that is what we should hope for. Big challenges are an incredible opportunity for personal growth and give us the chance to take our lives to a new level. It is not so much what has happened to us but how we deal with it that defines the calibre of the person we become.

Adversity is not something to fear. We like to have heroes, and the people who have faced the most difficult challenges are some of the most inspirational in society today. We don't so much celebrate their peak achievements as connect to their grit, determination and ability to rise from the bottom. The lower the lows, the more we appreciate the highs. It is the journey and not the destination that makes us admire them.

My aim in writing this book is to tell my personal story and share the mindset tools that I have honed along the way, so you can learn from them. Again, it is in the evolution that the lessons can be learned, and I am still a work in progress.

I have developed what I affectionately call my Ten Magical Mindset Rules, each of which forms the basis of a chapter in this book. I have always wanted to get my thoughts on paper in a meaningful way that could help others, and by a strange stroke of 'luck' I had a two-month stay in hospital in spring 2017 that got me started.

My challenges have made me who I am, but it hasn't been a solo effort. So many people have inspired and helped me on my journey, many of whom you will meet in this book. My burning desire is to pass on what I have learned, so I hope that everyone will find at least one 'Aha!' moment that sets them on their own path to acceptance and personal growth. Let's stay upbeat together!

CHAPTER 1

Your Diagnosis Does Not Define You

Everything can be taken from a man but one thing: the last of the human freedoms – to choose one's attitude in any given set of circumstances, to choose one's own way.

VIKTOR FRANKL

I have always known that my heart was different.

I was born on 22 October 1972, six weeks premature and weighing a tiny four pounds. It wasn't until I was six months old, during a doctor's visit for a chest infection, that somebody noted I had a heart murmur. Subsequent tests showed that I had a hole in the atrial septum, the division between the two upper heart chambers, and a stenosed (narrowed) pulmonary valve in the artery between the heart and lungs.

I am certainly blessed to have been born when I was. With paediatric heart surgery being in its infancy, even ten years earlier the outcome might have been very different. In spite of my parents' best efforts, I didn't thrive physically as a child. I had an incredibly happy childhood, but my early life was peppered with more than my share of chest infections and visits to doctors and hospitals. I don't recollect viewing myself as a 'sick' child, and this is testament to my parents, who never allowed me to feel physically inferior and did their best to treat me like a normal kid.

Perhaps the only visible indicator that I was different was my below-average height and body weight, which became more noticeable as I got older. I can only guess that my low body weight was a topic of discussion at my hospital appointments, as my diaries from the time reveal that I had started regularly writing down my weight. The earliest measurement I can find is from 6 April 1982: three stone and four pounds – almost two stone less than I should have been.

We moved to Cornwall when I was four years old, and my care was then spread between hospitals in Plymouth and Bristol. The NHS was not as 'joined up' as it is today, and it is easy to see from my medical notes the differing advice my parents were given and how strongly they had to advocate for my care. Getting my various doctors to agree on a plan of action wasn't straightforward, and I didn't have my first big surgery until 20 May 1982, when I was nearly 10 years old. The hole was repaired with a tissue patch (I made a joke at the time that it had been filled with Kleenex), and the valve was widened and repaired to improve the blood flow.

In the months running up to this surgery, for the first time in my life I started to feel that I was being singled out as different. I have clear recollections of being forced to sit at the side in PE class and watch, rather than take part. I don't know whether this was at my parents' request or the whim of the teachers, but it certainly planted the seed in my mind that I didn't like to be treated differently or have people make assumptions about my capabilities. Those feelings dramatically shaped my core values and attitude as I got older.

As was common with most early heart surgery, I spent many weeks in hospital and then a further four months at home recuperating. My parents had deliberately scheduled the operation to allow me time to recover over the summer holidays, meaning that I missed very little schooling. On my return I was something of a celebrity, with everyone bringing me gifts and wanting to see my scar. I didn't mind, and it was even fun for a while to feel that I was special, but soon enough I just wanted to fit in and be a normal child again. Aside from regular hospital follow-up appointments, that's pretty much what happened.

My childhood experiences had left their mark psychologically, though: as I entered senior school, I started to accept, maybe even subconsciously, that I was physically inferior to my peers. After surgery I had a huge growth spurt, and I distinctly remember my father commenting that it was like I had been placed in some manure. Although I no longer looked ill, years of being surrounded by people who knew I had a heart problem had left me accepting that sporting achievement probably wouldn't be my thing. It wasn't until I was almost 20 that I decided to test my theory and I discovered how incorrect my assumptions had been.

I went to a good private girls' school where physical and academic prowess were both celebrated, yet I didn't really excel at either. My grades were almost certainly based on my affinity with the teacher rather than my aptitude for the subject, so they varied wildly throughout my school years. Everyone recognised that I had potential, yet the most frequent phrase in my annual reports appeared to be 'could do better'. The only subject where I excelled was English language, where I got great joy from writing my own stories.

I was painfully shy and fairly introverted, so it was incredibly fortunate that I went to a small school, where I was much less likely to be bullied or picked on. I made my own way, never being one of the popular children or having many friends. I discovered a love of sailing when I was in my early teens, and that brought me into contact with a bunch of people much older than me. In the sailing community I finally found a place where I fitted in, and since then a love of water sports has been an ongoing theme in my life.

One person in particular, Mark, took me under his wing, and we are still the best of friends over thirty years later. Mark is loyal and trustworthy, and he has proven to be the first person to step up whenever I have faced a crisis. I am an only child, so he is rather like the brother I never had.

What I lacked was a real sense of purpose or direction. When many of my friends were leaving school to study and become doctors, accountants, vets or pharmacists, I didn't really have much idea. I wrote secret plans about how I was going to buy a boat and sail around the world, but my father, a highly qualified engineer working in the management team of the nearby naval dockyard at Devonport, insisted that I must go to university. With a mediocre selection of A levels, I reluctantly made the decision to take a business studies degree in Southampton.

I thought that living near the sea would at least allow me to nurture my love of sailing, but in fact my increasing insecurities and low self-confidence meant that I felt isolated and spent a lot of my time locked away in my room. Coming from a small private school and a sheltered childhood into the big bad world, I was incredibly naive and didn't know how to fit in. I didn't relate to people of my own age, hated the feeling of losing control that came from drinking alcohol, and felt out of my depth in all social situations.

Looking back, I can see that my childhood illnesses, health condition and surgery had more impact than I realised. Part of me wanted to use it to single myself out as special in the hope that people would like me, yet I also wanted to distance myself from that part of my history. The truth was that I didn't really like myself, so this inner conflict just caused confusion.

I was evidently depressed, and I can clearly remember having thoughts about running away from it all, taking an overdose or harming myself to attract attention. Although I never acted on these ideas, I remember my university years as being very difficult. The irony is that while I was angry at the world for apparently not understanding me, the biggest issue was that I didn't understand myself!

A pivotal moment in my life took place during the third year of my sandwich degree, when I was working for a Southampton-based marine-electronics company. I started dating Doug, who was sixteen years my senior, American and the marketing director. It was my first serious relationship, and he took me out for nice meals, weekend trips to London and even on a sailing trip to Miami.

I was guarded, naive and certainly not arm-candy, but he must have seen a spark underneath my hard shell. He was highly motivated and driven to succeed, and observing his habits instilled in me a set of values that I have never forgotten. He somehow accepted me with all my neuroses, and perhaps recognised my desperate need to love and be loved.

I remember so clearly, after a particularly morose conversation (one of many, I am sure), Doug said to me 'I love you very much, but I just don't want to be around you when you are like this' … and walked out of the door. At first, I was shocked and hurt, as I had been expecting him to feel sorry for me and validate my feelings. His response left me feeling I had been rejected. I felt sorry for myself for quite some time, seeking to justify why I had acted as I did, but after the anger and resentment had passed I started to wonder if he was right.

Was I putting on a negative persona to seek attention and make myself feel loved?

- Was it reasonable for me to feel this way?
- Could I start to view my life and its challenges differently?
- What kind of person might I be if I stopped wallowing in self-pity?
- Could I replace those negative emotions with something more positive, or at least neutral?
- What beliefs about my life would I have to change if I was to be happy?

Our relationship only lasted for about six months, until he returned to the USA. Although I followed him the next summer and spent several months living in Seattle, not surprisingly, things went no further. That might have been the signal for me to go off the rails again, but Doug had planted the seed that I had more control over my emotions than I thought: my state of mind was a choice.

I realised that I had to take ownership of what I achieved in my life and change my internal dialogue, or the voice in my head, so that I was no longer viewing myself as a victim. My mistake had been to blame (sometimes unconsciously) my heart condition for many of the difficulties in my life, and to use it as an excuse for not being and doing more. By giving it so much power, I had surrendered my ability to move on.

Doug introduced me to the book *Man's Search for Meaning*, by Austrian psychiatrist Viktor Frankl, first published in 1946, which detailed his experiences in the concentration camps. His book is filled with profound realisations and quotes – one of my favourites appears at the beginning of this chapter. Whether through reading the self-help books that Doug had on his shelves or by being inspired to follow his daily example of leading a life of purpose, I started to view my situation differently.

Having taken a good hard look at my mindset, my outlook and the person I wanted to be, I slowly transformed myself into a different person. As I started to take responsibility for all aspects of my life, my optimism and joy returned. I still hadn't found my real life's purpose, but I was certainly healthier and more content. My final year at university was much happier – although I still didn't thrive, I began to see that I had far more influence over the direction of my life than I thought. I started to become the driver in my life, not simply a passenger.

Shattered vase theory

In his book *What Doesn't Kill Us: A Guide to Overcoming Adversity and Moving Forward*, Professor Stephen Joseph discusses a metaphor he calls 'shattered vase theory'. In it he notes that if someone were to knock a precious vase from a table and it sustained little damage, they should be able to make an almost invisible repair. This represents a small but surmountable challenge, which does not have a significant impact on our lives.

On the other hand, if the vase shattered, it would likely be impossible to rebuild it with any strength. Attempts to do so would always leave obvious chips, cracks and lines of glue, and there would be ongoing weaknesses. This represents a significant trauma, which forces us to reconsider many of our assumptions about ourselves, our view of the world and how we fit in. Even if we can rebuild ourselves, trying desperately to be the person we were before will leave us vulnerable and prone to breaking again in the future.

The final option is to take the fragments, accept that the vase is broken beyond repair, and use the pieces to form a new and perhaps more beautiful object, such as a mural. In that way we can take the best of what remains of our sense of self, incorporate what we have learned, and use it as the foundation for a new and hopefully improved identity. Being forced to let go of our old beliefs and habits can be particularly painful. It can take months or even years to accept those changes and then grow from the adversity. Support from other people can help us through that process.

It seems remarkable to me now that Doug had such a profound influence on my life despite being part of it for such a short time. We never know how our interactions with others, no matter how brief, can change the course of a life. Doug certainly did that for me.

Doug had another life-changing effect on me, which I know he would not have appreciated at the time. He was a keen runner and triathlete, and while we were living together he frequently took himself off to do evening and weekend races. I never went with him, but it did give me the idea that running might be a way to take control of my expanding waistline. I certainly wasn't fat, but I had reached the heaviest I have ever been, and lack of exercise wasn't helping.

Up until this point, I had never tried to pursue any athletic endeavours. When I started out, I was desperately slow and unsure of how my body would cope. As my fitness levels improved, I began to wonder if my poor capabilities were more of an assumption than a reality. There was certainly no need to hang on to the 'sick girl' crutch any longer. It wasn't part of my new identity and I wanted to leave it, and the weakness it signalled, behind.

After some consistent training, it turned out that I was more capable than I thought. I certainly wasn't fast or genetically gifted, but as the length of my runs increased, my confidence grew. I went from being someone who had written herself off to being a person who wanted to be more active and push her boundaries. It turned out that physical expression was a good way to do this, and as almost nobody in my social circle knew my heart history any more, it was an entirely level playing field.

As far as I was concerned, my health problems were all behind me so I had little to fear. I had started to find excuses not to attend my annual cardiology follow-up appointments, as they just acted as an unwanted reminder that my heart was not normal. I felt invincible. Whether I just had assumed it or was told, I believed that no further intervention would ever be necessary.

At my last cardiology appointment in 1994, I mentioned to my consultant of many years that I had taken up running and wanted to check that this was OK. His response, which to me now seems entirely reasonable, was that it would be fine 'providing I didn't want to run marathons'. In case you haven't guessed it by now, that was like a red rag to a bull, and it precipitated my journey into endurance sports, marathons and beyond!

My irritation with his response – with its reminder that I hadn't fully escaped my past – meant that I deliberately dropped out of any follow-up care. That remained the case for the next eleven years. On graduation, I went to live in America temporarily while I figured out what to do next in life. The fact that I stayed there for nine years tells you that I found a country, friends and a lifestyle that I loved.

The decision to move to America was interesting. Until then I had rarely travelled out of the UK, let alone for an extended period. My new-found self-confidence had left me far more prepared to push my boundaries, and I was less fearful of making 'bad' decisions. I also stopped allowing myself to feel regret, and instead saw every life decision as either positive or a learning experience. I was testing my wings to see how far I could fly.

The year-round Florida sunshine and outdoor life led me into competitive running and, ultimately, long-distance triathlon. I became reasonably successful, training for between ten and twenty hours every week, racing most weekends and regularly winning prizes. Swimming, cycling and running formed a huge part of my identity and social circle, often to the detriment of everything else.

I have often wondered if I would have been so driven to challenge myself physically had it not been for my heart history. Part of me has always wanted to prove to others, and perhaps most importantly myself, that I am OK and that nothing is going to hold me back. I refuse to feel sorry for myself or to accept that I am in any way inferior. I would bet that many others who face significant medical adversity feel the same overwhelming need to prove they are invincible, and, in many respects, I don't think that's a bad thing.

My love of endurance athletics led me naturally into qualifying as a personal trainer and triathlon coach. I wasn't that good at marketing my services, though, and instead made most of my living running a computer servicing business. A few days after arriving in Florida, while working for a giant store selling new and used boating equipment, I had been introduced to a fellow Englishman called James. Rather like Doug and Mark, James has had a massive influence on the direction of my life, and although thousands of miles now separate us, I am proud to still call him one of my best friends.

James ran a successful computer business, and he took me under his wing and helped me to learn new skills. Much of our work was done either overnight or in the peak of the day, which left me plenty of time to go cycling, swimming and running during the cooler hours (only foolish people exercise during the extreme daytime humidity in Florida). My relationship with James quickly morphed from professional to personal, and I spent most of the nine years I was in Fort Lauderdale living under his roof. I am forever grateful for the security and encouragement he offered, and he continues to be one of my greatest supporters to this day.

Everything was about to change. One morning in September 1999, James woke me up to tell me that Mum had called to say that Dad had died of a massive heart attack the night before. He was only 55. Out of the blue, another pivotal moment in my life had occurred. It is said that the loss of a parent makes us question our place in the world, and although my relationship with my dad had been strained at times and I never felt I could measure up to his expectations, I miss him as much now as I did then.

I hit autopilot, booked a flight back to the UK, and spent the next few months helping my mum with the funeral and trying to rebuild her life. I felt strongly that my home was in Florida, so that December she returned there with me and spent the winter away from the miserable English weather.

My dad's untimely death was yet another reminder of the fragility of life and the importance of living for today. As much as I loved Florida and the life I had built for myself, I started to feel detached, so in 2002 I decided to move home to be closer to Mum and what remained of my family. Little did I know how fortuitous this would be.

CHAPTER 2

Every Emotion Is Under Your Control – Always!

If you're pessimistic and against yourself the deck becomes too stacked – I implore all of you to choose optimism over pessimism and allow yourself to be your own biggest fan.

GARY VAYNERCHUK

Around 2001, while still living in Florida, I had started to experience increasingly frequent heart palpitations and a noticeable fall in exercise tolerance. Since I was nearing 30, I attributed these issues to getting older, but on reflection I should have recognised that something was wrong.

I took my declining race performance and results as a signal to train harder, but it seemed that no matter what I did I wasn't as successful as before. I had managed to cover up the health concerns of my childhood by pretending that part of my history didn't exist. Doubtless that also motivated me to become such a dedicated athlete, as if by doing this I could prove to myself that I was all right. As things declined, I was having to face an unwanted reality – but even then, I buried my head in the sand and tried to carry on as before.

It wasn't until soon after my return to the UK that things came to a head. Slightly unsure of a career path, and still craving my Florida life, I had taken an eighteen-month contract working in the civil service as an assistant farm inspector. Strange as that may sound, having grown up in the countryside I have a real affinity with rural life, and most of all I didn't want to find myself trapped behind a desk.

I loved the variety of my work and the outdoor life, but after a stressful few months commuting to an office in Exeter, fifty miles from home, my symptoms became increasingly bothersome. On several occasions I had to go to A&E with rhythm problems. After one scary weekend where I found myself crawling around the house because I felt dizzy every time I stood up, I went to my GP, who swiftly referred me to the hospital.

I saw several doctors, and it soon became clear that my issues were likely related to my childhood surgery. Ultimately, I fell back under the care of the same consultant I had last seen some eleven years earlier. I had to confess that I had naively chosen to stop attending my annual appointments, and I was now back in the system with the hope that he could help me.

What my parents and I had never been told, likely because the medical profession didn't know it themselves at the time, was that my childhood surgery was not a 'cure'. With significantly greater numbers of children with congenital heart defects now living into adulthood, the longer-term effects and possible complications are now better understood. In my case, the progressively worsening leakage of my pulmonary valve had put a lot of strain on the right side of my heart. It had grown as a result, becoming a larger but less efficient pumping chamber, and the stretched muscle was causing the rhythm problems, fatigue and breathlessness that I had been experiencing. This wasn't brilliant news, but I was more than a little relieved that I finally had some answers.

The only solution was going to be further open-heart surgery to replace my pulmonary valve. At first I was quite resistant to the idea because, apart from the increasing breathlessness and palpitations, I didn't feel that bad. Only now do I realise how much I was being affected. When we experience a slow decline in health rather than a sudden event, it is easy not to notice that it is happening. We adapt and our expectations of ourselves imperceptibly change. It is not until after treatment that we realise how bad things were.

The year I spent awaiting surgery was difficult. I felt relieved that the symptoms I was experiencing were not all in my head and that there was a solution, but I also felt a gnawing anxiety about the risks involved.

There were occasions when I was angry and resentful that life had thrown me this new and unwanted challenge. I questioned if there was anything I could have done to prevent it, or if the life choices I had made might have made my situation worse. Rationally, I knew that this was just part of the natural progression of my condition, but, particularly in the days following my new diagnosis, I was annoyed that my body was again letting me down.

All those fears of being perceived as weak, which I had hated as a child, resurfaced. Part of my reaction was to pretend that nothing was wrong and try to carry on as before. I immersed myself in my work and exercise routine, and unless you knew me well you wouldn't have recognised that anything was amiss.

During this period, having left the civil service, I took on a variety of agency jobs because I didn't want to have to explain my health situation to a new employer. It is hard to seek permanent employment when you know you are soon going to need three months off work. By coincidence, I settled into a temporary position as an X-ray clerk at Derriford Hospital in Plymouth – the very hospital where I was being treated.

It was a demanding role, zipping around the hospital trying to find the X-ray film packets for every patient on the orthopaedic outpatient clinic list. Some were in the film store, some still waiting to be reported, others on a ward and a fair few 'lost' in various consultants' offices. There was a computerised tracking system, but it relied on people taking the time to note that they had moved the packets, something that was often overlooked. To find them, you needed lateral thinking, intuition and dogged determination!

Being on my feet for most of the day was hard work. I had to travel between levels 3, 6, 10 and 11, and I didn't have time to wait for the lift so I usually took the stairs. I walked miles every day, often with piles of heavy X-ray films under my arm. I viewed the metal trolley I was supposed to use as more of a speed handicap than a useful asset.

I became adept at finding the missing films, and I enjoyed the sense that I was doing my bit to make another patient's journey more positive. I believe in karma: I feel strongly that if I do my best to help others, reciprocal good will come into my life or that of someone I love. I can't prove my theory, but I prefer to view the world in that way.

I was aware that some consultants would refuse to see a patient if the films were not viewable in the clinic. Much as I understood that rationale, it acted as a clear motivator to do the best job I could. Luckily, films are now stored digitally so the days of running around a hospital trying to track down a physical film packet are long gone.

I have always been goal-orientated, and I gained a great deal of personal satisfaction from seeing a clinic list and methodically crossing off the patients' files as I found them. Unfortunately, my perfectionist nature also means that I hate not being successful, so the fact that some of the X-ray packets just couldn't be found was quite stressful for me. I rarely sat down, constantly rushed around the hospital, and often took my lunch break on the hop.

Although the job kept me fit, I remember on one occasion climbing the stairs and being so out of breath and dizzy that I couldn't get the stairwell door open with people coming up behind me. A doctor, noticing my condition, seemed genuinely concerned that I must sit down and kept asking 'Are you sure you're OK?' I remember assuring him that I was, when it wouldn't have taken a medical professional to see that I wasn't!

Yet again, I was trying to prove to myself that I was unstoppable and that I wouldn't let this setback beat me. Behind the facade, I was really scared. In the space of a few years I had gone from being Beth the super-fit athlete to someone who struggled going up a flight of stairs. I was fearful that people would again start to see me as broken or someone to be pitied. I didn't want people's perceptions of me to change, but perhaps most of all I worried that I was having to adjust my own feelings about how I fitted into the world. If I wasn't who I had been before, who was I now?

I started to mourn for my old life and crave its return, and I had to suppress a desire to run back to the USA and pretend this wasn't happening. My memories of my first surgery were ill-defined, and I associated it with having more of a psychological impact than a physical one. Now my physical capacity was being challenged, and that was having a negative effect on my mental health. My self-confidence took a real knock as I found my chosen identity being slowly peeled away, rather like the layers of an onion.

I usually chose not to share my worries with others, and instead spent time alone processing my thoughts and feelings as a way of coming to terms with them. I always came back to the idea that I had been here before, medical science had progressed, and if I did nothing then my quality of life would continue to decline. Ultimately, I would die needlessly.

Having now spent many years studying how to overcome trauma, I recognise that the coping strategies I instinctively adopted were those that experts recommended to someone in my position. I kept up with as many of my normal habits and routines as I could. It is easy, when facing a dramatic life event, to withdraw and stop doing the things that used to make us feel fulfilled. Many people suggested that I should stop work and take more time to relax – yet that regular routine and sense of normality was exactly what I needed.

I continued to work full time until a week before my surgery, mainly because I didn't want to have too much time to dwell on the 'what ifs' of my situation. I could go to work and largely forget my worries, which wasn't so easy when I was alone at home. Working also forced me to maintain my social circle and stay engaged with the people around me. I am far from a naturally gregarious person, and at times of stress I have a strong instinct to withdraw. Had I not been going to work, I would probably have spent my days at home, brooding on my situation and sliding back into that cycle of self-pity and depression.

I am still great friends with a few of my colleagues from this period, and their support was pivotal in giving me strength. I am fiercely independent, so to admit that I needed help was incredibly hard. My instinct was to shut people out, and I can only guess that at times I came across as aloof or even resentful of people's genuine attempts to make my life easier. I shunned any suggested allowances, as they only served to make me feel inferior. I needed to prove to everyone else, and to myself, that I could cope.

Although my arrhythmias continued to plague me and my capacity for exercise reduced further, I did my utmost to maintain my fitness. That image of fitness and health was still very much a part of my identity, and sticking to my routine gave me a sense of control that was otherwise lacking in my life. I was still going to the gym most mornings before work, and I even ran a reasonable half-marathon about six weeks before my operation. I was tired beyond measure, but I firmly believe that the efforts I made before surgery had a massive influence on the speed with which I recovered.

I also started paying more attention to nutrition. My diet is usually fairly healthy, but it was easy to slide into seeking comfort food to suppress my worries and make me superficially happy. I had to remind myself that the food I ate was fuel for my body, and I needed to go into this surgery feeling as strong as I could. Eating junk might make me feel satisfied in the short term, but it wouldn't give my body the nutrients it needed to rest and repair. Equally, poor nutrition just made me feel bad, lacking in energy and cross with myself, which exacerbated any negative feelings I was having.

About eight months into my agency role, my supervisor at the hospital told me that they were going to advertise my job. It had been impossible to keep my upcoming surgery a secret from everyone, but when asked if I was going to apply for the position, I told her that I was not. I felt uncomfortable doing so with the knowledge that I was likely to be on sick leave for many months. I was also mindful that I had only ever seen this job as temporary, while I decided what to do next in life. Although a permanent role would give me the benefits of job security and sick pay, it didn't seem right to take it. Despite my protests, my supervisor assured me that if I were to apply I would stand a good chance of getting the job – and that turned out to be the case.

Working at the hospital was rather fortunate. Scheduling tests and appointments was much easier, I often bumped into members of my medical team around the hospital, and everything seemed to happen a little more efficiently. I already knew that my local hospital in Plymouth would not be able to carry out my surgery, so I was referred to the specialist congenital heart centre in Bristol. My wonderful consultant there was a keen athlete himself, so we had an instant connection. He knew how badly I wanted to keep up my athletic lifestyle, and he did his best to allay my fears.

I knew I was doing the right thing, and as the date of my operation got closer I became increasingly confident about what lay ahead.

I certainly had some sleepless nights, which led to me spending a lot of time online reading all the medical research I could find on surgical risks, complications and outcomes. That knowledge acted as a comfort: I regained my sense of control over what was going to happen, and I was at peace with my choices. Of course, I knew that there was a chance I could die, but the possibility was small enough not to bother me. I was far more concerned about how quickly I would be able to regain my fitness and get back to the lifestyle I enjoyed.

I chose to focus my thoughts on how much better I would feel after the surgery. I expected my physical fitness to increase, maybe even beyond what I had previously been able to achieve. I was also keen to get the surgery over with, so I could get out of what felt like a holding pen and move on with my life.

I realised that I had a choice: I could allow my fear and worry to consume me, or I could see this obstacle as an opportunity for growth. I rationalised that I had probably spent much of the previous twenty-three years with a dodgy heart valve, so I expected to recover to be physically more able. Although that turned out not to be the case exactly, I am certain that my positivity contributed to things going smoothly before and after surgery.

The hero's journey

It was around this time that I began studying the stories of others who had overcome trauma and adversity. I learned of the writings of Joseph Campbell, an early twentieth-century mythologist, who detailed the stages of a hero's journey in his book *The Hero with a Thousand Faces*. The hero's journey is a cycle, where a person with an ordinary life is forced to take a path on which they face significant challenges. They seek help from a mentor, reach a major crisis point and face a physical or metaphorical battle. When they come out the other side, they return to some aspects of their earlier life, but they are stronger and more resilient.

If we look at many bestselling books and movies, such as *The Lord of The Rings*, *Harry Potter* or *Star Wars*, we can identify aspects of the hero's journey in them. It is easy to believe that stories bear no relationship to real life, yet we all must overcome adversity of some sort in our lives. It is doubtful that this alone makes our life worthy of a movie franchise, but I believe that we are all heroes in our own way. Medical adversity sets us off on a journey we didn't want or plan to go on, into uncharted waters and with an uncertain outcome. Whether we sink or swim often comes down to resilience and strength of character.

I have added my own interpretation of the stages of the hero's journey, specifically in the context of medical adversity:

1. Introduction to the hero's world. This is you, in your normal life. Who are you? What are your beliefs? What defines your character?
2. Call to action. A big medical challenge or diagnosis. The moment when you know that things are going to change and your life will never be the same.
3. Crossing the threshold. Loss of identity, isolation, uncertainty, fear and denial.
4. Meet the mentor. We can't do it alone – we all need help. Often this is a person or people in the medical profession, but it could be a family member or great friend who inspires you, guides you and helps you on your journey.
5. First challenge. Facing up to our fears. Learning about and accepting a treatment plan. Surrendering some control.
6. Temptation. Self-doubt.
7. Dark inner moment. A low point. Despair.
8. The final battle. Perhaps an operation or invasive treatment.
9. The return home. Rebuilding yourself – not as the same person, but better than before. You feel stronger and more able to face the future.

It is interesting that the typical hero's journey seems to be linear. In my own experience of medical adversity, though, things were not so well defined. It may well be that we face multiple challenges and dark moments before we reach that return or acceptance in our life. What the hero's journey highlights for me is that it is an evolutionary process, and that holding on tight to our old identity doesn't work. If we are to move on emotionally, we must be prepared to let go of what may seem comfortable but is no longer beneficial. True personal growth only occurs when we accept that loss and incorporate the change into our new life story.

I love the premise that significant adversity can be a catalyst for growth, rather than something that automatically has negative consequences. It is often people who have overcome the biggest challenges who go on to achieve remarkable things. If Viktor Frankl could somehow find benefit in his incarceration and solitary confinement at Auschwitz, there is hope for us all.

The Chinese symbol for a crisis is a combination of the symbols for danger and opportunity, signalling that there are positives and negatives to be found in any experience. Even the bleakest situation has an 'up' side. It is how we categorise an experience that counts; one person might see it as a minor inconvenience and another may view it as a dramatic event.

The truth is that bad things happen to good people. We may not have much control over what happens to us, but we can decide how we react. It can be beneficial to find role models who have found themselves in similar situations and try to understand what they did to rise above their adversity. We all love media stories about 'normal' people who achieve remarkable things despite overwhelming odds – we feel hope and find inspiration in the strength of the human spirit.

These things also remind us of the fragility and randomness of life. Every day, people get diagnosed with cancer, suffer life-changing injuries, have car accidents, get hurt in terrorist attacks, and a whole host of other misfortunes that they do not deserve and cannot possibly foresee. We can go through life fearing the onset of such trauma, or we can decide to celebrate the here and now and make the most of life.

CHAPTER 3

Focus On The Parts Of Life You Can Control

Experience is not what happens to you; it's what you do with what happens to you.

ALDOUS HUXLEY

In August 2005, it was with a sense of relief that I was admitted to the Bristol Royal Infirmary for my surgery. I was physically and psychologically prepared – if anything, I was impatient to get this major hurdle over with so I could begin the rebuilding process.

When I wasn't having my pre-op checks, I read to keep my mind occupied. I had a pile of magazines with me – most of them related to triathlons or running. I was quite aware of how incongruous that must have seemed to the other patients on the ward, most of whom were at least thirty years older than me.

I spent the night in a bay with three older ladies, and I distinctly remember trying to distract myself by sharing stories, laughing and joking. I was woken early in the morning and taken to a private room, where I had the obligatory shower in Hibiscrub –

an antibacterial disinfectant solution that smells vile and wouldn't pass as a body wash in the worst of hotels.

I dressed myself in a fetching surgical gown, and after being given a pre-med to help me relax, I was left to sleep. Unfortunately, the surgery before mine over-ran and the hours ticked by, so I was very much 'with it' by the time the porters came to take me to theatre. Humour is one of my main coping mechanisms when I'm scared, so I am sure that I cracked a joke or two while the anaesthetist did his thing. I was connected to various monitors, and the sleepy elixir trickled into my veins.

My next recollection was coming round in the intensive care unit. Someone was asking me if I wanted the breathing tube to be taken out. I nodded approval before lapsing again into sleep. Unfortunately, my lasting memories of the next few hours are not of some restful tropical beach but of retching repeatedly, something I now know to be an after-effect of the morphine I was given during and after the op. If you have ever tried being repeatedly sick with your sternum newly cut and wired back together, you will know that it is not to be recommended.

The sickness was unrelenting, no matter what anti-emetics were administered, and I overheard someone saying that a nurse had been sent to the oncology ward for something stronger. Most worryingly, my blood pressure and heart rate became dangerously low, and I was aware that at one point defibrillator pads were attached to my chest in case my heart stopped.

Thankfully, once the immediate crisis had passed, things quickly improved. I made the step down to the high dependency unit and, once a bed became available a few days later, back to the ward. Over a period of days, I was slowly weaned off the drugs and the number of tubes, wires and drains poking out of my body was reduced.

What shocked me was how weak I felt. I was painfully aware of the insult my body had received, but I had a hard time processing why I wasn't just going to get back to normal within a few days.

I hit a real low point one morning, when I found that I didn't have the strength to move my breakfast table towards me. Whether it was from pure frustration, the after-effects of the anaesthetic or a combination of both, I clearly remember sitting back in the chair and sobbing.

Once I had recovered my composure, I realised that I had a choice. I could continue to be Beth, the victim of her circumstances who was forever using them as an excuse, or I could pick myself up, dust off my pride and decide to become the best version of me that I could. I started my quest soon after, standing up and shuffling to the end of the bed and back. A few hours later when I tried again, I made it to the end of the bay; next time, to the nurse's station. I soon discovered that it was a circular ward and if I kept walking I would end up back where I started. Then there was no stopping me.

Over a few days I began to build up my laps, competing with myself to go a little further each time. This was quite unlike any athletics training I had done before, but the method of slow progress was the same. The feelings of achievement acted as a positive motivator and my confidence grew.

People often ask how I managed to cope so well with my surgery and its aftermath. I think that my early life experiences helped, as I already knew that I could put myself back together if I could take control of my thought processes. Although I avoided them at times, I spent huge chunks of time deliberately facing up to my fears, deciding which aspects I could control and which I could not.

I forced myself to engage with my current situation, accepting my limitations while trying to find practical solutions to the things I could change. I have always been a deep thinker – sometimes this has led to paralysing over-analysis, but this time it worked in my favour. I rationalised that although I couldn't have full control over my medical status, I still had a big say in how I perceived what was happening to me and what I did with that information.

My state of mind – whether happy, sad, irritable, calm, accepting or combative – was something that only I could influence. No matter what other dignity or control I had to relinquish, I found a great deal of solace in realising that I still had the power to make that decision.

Living with my heart condition in this crisis period certainly stripped away much of my independence and confidence, and at times my self-esteem suffered. Yet I knew that if I was less anxious about the areas of my life I couldn't directly influence, I would have more resources to focus on those I could. My best advice is not to put emotional energy into things you can't change.

Acceptance is a vital trait for anyone facing a significant trauma. Until this setback, though, I believed I had to accept all aspects of my situation, without question. I now know that this is not the case, and to accept blindly lessened my ability to overcome it. I had to use my judgement to tease out the aspects I could change and those I couldn't. Fretting about things I couldn't change was wasted emotion, and worse still it weakened my ability to stay positive.

It is almost like I had a 'coping bucket', where the life challenges flowed in from the top and out through a hole in the bottom where I could process them. If I allowed too many negative thoughts to build up, the contents of the bucket overflowed and I fell into crisis. On the other hand, if I dealt with my fears, kept perspective, maintained healthy habits and never lost hope, I was far more able to cope with what was happening to me.

I discovered that it was still important to acknowledge how I was feeling, but I could simply observe those emotions, rather like a bystander, instead of allowing them to take over my mind. If I didn't deal with negative thoughts, they had the power to take on a life of their own, where they could fester and grow into something much bigger. I certainly had my moments of fear and worry, but I managed to maintain a balance with optimism and hope.

Learned helplessness

American psychologist Martin Seligman is a world-renowned researcher in the field of positive psychology and resilience. He is also the author of several amazing books, such as *Learned Optimism: How to Change Your Mind and Your Life* (2006). Seligman coined the term 'learned helplessness' to describe what happens when people falsely assume that because of a previous experience, an aspect of their future is inescapable. An example in my case is my assumption that because I had not been a sporty child due to my heart condition I could never become an athlete, even after I had surgery that improved my health. I lacked the confidence to even test things out until someone else inspired me to question my belief.

Seligman also studied why people can respond differently to similar traumatic events depending on how they choose to perceive them. He called this a person's 'explanatory style' and detailed three attributes of this. The first is 'permanence' ('I have no ability to ever change this situation' versus 'This may be the situation right now, but it will get better'), the second is 'personal' ('It is all my fault' versus 'Other factors had an influence') and the third is 'pervasiveness' ('It is going to have a negative effect on the rest of my life' versus 'It changes some things but not everything').

Imagine what my recovery would have been like if, after my second surgery, I convinced myself that I could have prevented it if I had looked after myself better, that it was going to cost me my chosen career and, by default, my ability to earn a decent living, and that now I would never be able to enjoy exercise again!

We have all been victims of that pessimistic thinking at some point. I also recognise that once you fall into a cycle of negative thinking, it can be very hard to break. I believe that a little wallowing in self-pity is not unhealthy and may even allow us to work through the worse-case scenarios, but if we allow that situation to continue it robs us of our future happiness.

Other than my mum, my biggest rock in this period was Rachel, a senior physiotherapist who became my firmest friend soon after I started working at Derriford Hospital. Rachel is the type of person you cannot help but admire – she's physically athletic and strong, funny, generous with her time, talented at her job, has boundless energy and a zest for life, is genuinely interested in people and makes the most of every opportunity.

I am mediocre at best in many of those areas, yet our friendship endures. Rachel understands my character, and although she is fiercely independent herself, I can rely on her to drop everything (without asking) and turn up in any moment of need. Rachel acted as the go-between, keeping my colleagues up to date with my progress. She also helped me to stay active before and after my operation, meeting me at the gym and getting me out and about even when I didn't feel like it. I am thankful that Rachel was, and still is, a constant in my life.

After my experience with morphine, pain management was an issue. I was reluctant to take anything for fear the nausea would return. Aside from the obvious pain in my sternum, my upper back, neck and shoulders were in agony. I couldn't get comfortable whether I was lying down, sitting or standing. It felt like somebody had torn a vertical strip out of my chest, opened my ribcage like a book, messed about with the contents, and then somehow yanked everything back together... which I suppose in essence they had!

Worst of all, my chin felt like it had been pulled towards my breastbone so that I couldn't look ahead – I could only see where I was going by leaning backward. It was awkward and uncomfortable. Even my surgeon, when he found me wandering around the ward several days later, looked a little surprised by my strange posture and apologised, not that he had any reason to do so.

As physically painful as it was, none of that mattered because I was still very much alive and ready to begin the rebuilding process. It took me three or four months of almost hourly stretching to relieve the tightened tissues so I could look straight ahead. Longest to recover was my upper back, which plagued me for almost a year until I found a sympathetic massage therapist who helped me to sort it out.

I believe my desire to aid my own recovery and be a star patient helped make sure that I was discharged from hospital just six days after surgery. If it hadn't been for some fluctuations in my potassium levels, I would have been discharged even sooner. My mum came to collect me and I spent the car journey from Bristol back to Cornwall with a pillow between my chest and the seatbelt to avoid discomfort.

I wasn't allowed to drive for six weeks after surgery, as if I had an accident and my chest hit the steering wheel this could seriously injure my damaged ribcage. Until then, I happily went to live with my mum. This was a blessing in many respects. Firstly, her cooking is awesome, unlike mine, and I really didn't have the energy to stand for long periods of time. If I had been living on my own, it would have been easy to resort to eating less wholesome convenience food.

Secondly, I live in the depths of the Cornish countryside far away from any bus route, so without being able to drive I would have been virtually housebound. Thirdly, Mum is the happy owner of an amazing Tempurpedic foam mattress and fully adjustable bed, which made it possible for me to find a somewhat comfortable sleeping position. Nothing quite prepares you for the difficulties in performing tasks that you normally take for granted, from rolling over in bed to taking a shower and getting dressed.

Everything seemed to take twice as long and involve some degree of discomfort.

As my recovery continued, I started to keep a detailed diary showing how far I had walked, my visits to the gym, and any other notable achievements for the day. That turned out to be one of the best motivational tools I had. It helped to stay positive on days when I started to lose confidence or feel despondent about the speed of my progress. I could look back and see how far I had come since my days in the intensive care unit and how my endurance was improving as the weeks went by.

I had to deal with the inevitable ups and downs in energy levels, as well as an overwhelming tiredness that seemed to strike without reason. I had always been good at listening to my body's signals about what it needs, but that had been tempered by my desire to master and control it. Now I was forced to accept that I needed time to physically heal, and allowing extra rest was the only way to do this.

Without the need to wake early each day to go to work, it would have been easy to while away my nights watching TV or browsing the internet, but I stuck to my 10pm lights out routine. Sleep is when our body and mind have time to rest and repair. I also recognised that I needed extra physical and emotional strength to recover from the stress I had been under, so I knew that I couldn't afford to get tired and deplete my reserves. More sleep, not less, was a big factor in accelerating my recovery.

It was interesting that as I regained mastery of my body, I grew in mental strength too. I went from being hyper-aware of every potential symptom to having a growing confidence that I was going to be OK. There were good days and bad, and progress was never linear, but the overall trajectory was definitely up.

CHAPTER 4

Learn From The Past, Look To The Future

Every problem has in it the seeds of its own solution. If you don't have any problems, you don't get any seeds.

NORMAN VINCENT PEALE

I was amazed by how much my recovery seemed to accelerate once I was away from the incessant hospital noise and able to get a full night's sleep. With good food and gentle daily exercise, I started taking leaps and bounds. Looking back at my exercise log, I can see that just three weeks after surgery I ran for 45 minutes (4.5 miles), biked in the gym for 45 minutes (14.5 miles) and swam 1,000 metres (40 lengths). I was incredibly determined to get back to triathlon, and I took part in a small local event at the gym just six weeks after surgery.

Part of my impatience came from my desire to distance myself from what had happened, and it wasn't until several months later that the full psychological impact became apparent. I wouldn't say that I was depressed, but the initial euphoria of having survived and the positive feelings I had during the first few months of my recovery had certainly worn off. I have since read several articles and studies about 'post-op blues' and I can see that it is something that many people experience.

I hadn't allowed myself the time to fully process my feelings as I went into the operation, and I had focused my efforts deliberately on my work and exercise regime. There was an element of denial about my longer-term health, which, ultimately, I had to face up to. As my initial super-fast recovery merged into a normal day-to-day routine, I became increasingly frustrated that I still seemed to have restrictions. My resting heart rate was still a good ten or fifteen beats higher than it had been before surgery, and my breathlessness, although better, was not resolved.

I had placed so much pressure on myself to have a remarkable recovery that the stark reality of my ongoing struggles was rather hard to take. I wanted to get on with my life as if nothing had happened, but there were indications everywhere that it had.

I started to realise that I was different, not just physically but mentally. I had been forced to question quite a few of my beliefs about who I was, what I stood for, and my expectations, hopes and dreams for the future. Although two years had passed since my return from America, this medical trauma had come on top of the death of my father, the failure of my marriage, my relocation, buying a home, attempts to become financially independent again and the slow stripping away of my 'athlete' identity.

I was clinging to aspects of my old life, but I felt like a rudderless ship at the whim of the winds and currents. Once again, I was at a crossroads in my life, but I had a much better toolbox than I did in my early twenties. Given plenty of thinking time to work through my emotions and feelings, I started to feel ready to move on with my life. I became determined that this surgery would be a catalyst for growth and that I would come back stronger and more resilient.

I also realised that I had been so focused on getting over my operation and back to my old life that I had forgotten how to do the things that brought me joy. I had lost myself in the day-to-day challenges, and perhaps subconsciously I felt that I didn't deserve to be happy any more. When survival was my focus, that was OK, but after that I knew just getting by was no longer enough.

I began to wonder if I was immersing myself in work not just as a distraction but also as a form of punishment. I felt annoyed that my body had let me down again, and I had lost trust in my own capabilities. The adversity I had faced had given me endless determination, but it also had the potential to steal my joy. I was so ready for everything to be a struggle that I couldn't relax and be objective about my future.

At first, I had to force myself to schedule fun events – to take a long solo ride on my bike, have dinner with my friends or buy tickets to a concert. Although I had always valued experiences more than possessions, I had to remind myself that it was still OK to have fun and that I didn't have to have any reason to do something other than the fact that it felt good.

Whenever I found myself sliding into a negative mindset about everything that had happened, I recognised that I had the power to turn things around if I kept a clear perspective. No matter what situation we find ourselves in, it is important to remember that there is always someone who is a lot worse off. I may have had some battle scars, but I was alive. Had I been born in a different country, I might not have had access to the wonderful medical services and support I had, and I probably wouldn't have made it out of adolescence. This latest episode could have been so much worse, and my overwhelming feelings were those of gratitude.

I chose to look at everything I had gained from my challenging health situation. I had built an incredible inner strength and an ability to master my own mind. I had met so many inspiring people from all walks of life, who had helped me to grow and develop. I had learned to look forward with optimism, rather than be held back by the past.

I acknowledged how fortunate I had been to have reached the ripe old age of 33, and how easily the situation could have been different. I felt more empathy for people who faced similar challenges, especially those of a medical nature. Most of all, I felt truly blessed to be alive and able to continue leaving my legacy. Far from holding me back, my difficulties had catapulted me forward.

Post-traumatic growth

A few years ago, I learned about 'post-traumatic growth', a term coined in the 1990s by Richard Tedeschi and Lawrence Calhoun at the University of North Carolina in Charlotte. They defined it as 'a positive change experienced as a result of the struggle with a major life crisis or traumatic event'. They published their findings in a 1996 article in *The Journal of Traumatic Stress*, entitled 'The Posttraumatic Growth Inventory: Measuring the positive legacy of trauma'.

The authors looked at evidence in previous scientific studies on the negative psychological effects of trauma. They found that, although trauma always resulted in some form of suffering, at least half of trauma survivors also reported benefits.

Tedeschi and Calhoun distilled their work into a 21-item post-traumatic growth inventory, dividing that growth into five main areas:

1. A desire to maximise potential and seek out new opportunities
2. An improved connection and relationship with others
3. A deeper sense of self-reliance and personal strength
4. A greater appreciation for life and its possibilities
5. A strengthening of spirituality or belief system

We can all grow after a traumatic event. That growth does not necessarily occur across the board – often, it happens in several specific areas where we were not as cognitively or emotionally developed before. Importantly, the trauma survivors who had the best coping strategies beforehand, or who did not perceive the event as being significant, tended to experience the least growth. In other words, if there is no challenge then positive change is less likely.

I believe that I have grown in all five of those main areas, and that process has continued with each successive challenge. Perhaps one of the biggest benefits of a major life-changing event is that it makes us re-evaluate our lives and what we want to achieve. It's like a metaphorical slap across the face, which brings about a period of heightened awareness and reflection. Without that impact, it is easy for us to stay in our comfort zone and for life to slip by.

On my return to work three months after surgery, the occupational health team insisted that I took on a more sedentary role. Although I had some incredibly supportive colleagues, I missed the autonomy and challenge of my old job. In the preceding few months, I had also started to acknowledge that it was not my destiny to be an X-ray clerk in the hospital and it was time to move on. I still wasn't entirely sure where my future lay, but I handed in my notice and enrolled on a four-month residential course in Bristol to re-qualify as a personal trainer.

My American certifications, although above the level I was going to study at, were not recognised in the UK, so the easiest choice was to start again. The old me would have seen this as a step backward and been frustrated that I had to spend money to go over old ground, but I chose to view it as another step towards a more fulfilling future. I felt drawn back into the world of fitness and health, and I had a strong feeling that it was part of my purpose in life.

I enjoyed everything about the course, and at last I could sense that I was on the right path. Over the next few years, I took more advanced qualifications, the most significant of which led me towards working with people with long-term medical conditions, such as heart disease, lung conditions, cancer, diabetes and stroke. I could use my own experience to prove the virtues of regular exercise, not only in preventing illness in the first place but also in aiding recovery when a difficult diagnosis is made.

I knew first-hand how important it was to use exercise as a way of taking back control, and how much that flow of endorphins raises our confidence and quality of life. What I didn't expect was how much the emotional support provided by group exercise could enhance recovery.

Lifelong illness often makes us feel singled out and misunderstood in society, maybe even by our own family. In group exercise with others who share something with our own life story, we can start to feel that we are not so alone. I remember with great fondness a group of women with breast cancer asking if they could use my private office to compare their scars, an opportunity that might not have arisen in most other environments.

Gentle exercise with others who have health conditions also allows us to realise that there is a lot of life still to be had beyond a diagnosis, and the diagnosis need not define everything about us. It puts our own situation into clear perspective. I can't tell you how many people have come to me after a class and relayed how grateful they were that they had their medical issues and not those of someone else in the group … and then to have that person say exactly the same in reverse!

I have also had the honour to meet a truly amazing group of people and to do my best to be a positive influence on part of their recovery. It has made my own struggles feel normal, and it has made me realise that there is no such thing as an easy life. While some of us are forced to deal with difficult medical situations, others have challenges with their finances, work, relationships, bereavement, addiction and so much more.

It can be easy to assume that because someone's outer persona looks as if they have everything figured out, they do not struggle with their own obstacles, insecurities and challenges. I have often found that the people with the hardest lives are some of the happiest and most grateful individuals I know.

Part of being alive means having to face difficult times, and we cannot avoid this no matter how much money, fame or optimism we have. We have all experienced upset and loss, when our lives have changed radically in a split second and without warning. I guarantee that there will be more of those moments on the way, and the only option is to deal with them as best we can. Some may say that is a pessimistic view, yet for me, acknowledging that there will be hard times ahead means I have less to fear. It is also a great reminder to make the most of the present moment.

My mindset is that no matter what happens in my life, I will find a way to make the most of it. The hardest times can be the most powerful in terms of turning us from regular to exceptional human beings. If we look at our modern-day heroes, we often find that they have faced great challenges, often more than once, and have come back stronger. We don't admire them for their best achievements, but for that story of challenge and regrowth.

I have often wondered if my own roller-coaster journey has been made easier by the fact that I have always known of my condition, so my identity has been built around it from the beginning. It is an interesting question, and I am slightly unsure of the answer. I recently saw a television show where a gentleman who had been blind since birth related that he thought his situation must be easier than that of someone who had lost their sight slowly or later in life, where they were painfully aware of what had been taken away.

The only thing I am sure of is that I will not live in fear of future loss. The medical and life challenges I have already had to overcome have made me the person I am, and I like to think that

I am a better human being because of them. I live in the present, choosing not to beat myself up about the mistakes I have made in the past or look too far into the future, with all its uncertainty.

Fear of the future can really hold us back if we are continually worrying about things that haven't happened yet, or instantly assuming the worst-case scenario when something does. Psychiatrists term this 'catastrophising' and view it as a form of anxiety or cognitive distortion, where we present a situation as considerably worse than it actually is.

I know that I have been a victim of this at times, and I think it can be particularly hard to control our anxiety, especially when we are living with a long-term health condition. We are naturally aware that things can go wrong at any minute, and those health challenges can be unpredictable. Yet there is no point in worrying about things that haven't happened yet, and perhaps never will.

There is a balance to be found. It is not necessarily a bad thing to consider all the possible outcomes when we face uncertainty, but I find it useful to grade each of them by their likelihood of occurring. In doing so, I can rationalise that the worst outcomes are unlikely to happen, and, more to the point, I would undoubtedly find a way to cope if they did.

I find it useful not to look too far into the future or to dwell on the past. In accepting my current reality, I am not surrendering my ability to shape my future life in a positive way, but I am conceding that the 'here and now' is the only place I have control.

I used to imagine how my life might look if I didn't have my heart condition, and then to paint it in a rather rose-tinted light. That is the ultimate in wasted time and emotion, when the reality is that I can only control what happens from this point onwards. I think that my decision not to allow negative emotions, such as resentment or anger, to linger in my thoughts, has been pivotal in how quickly I have bounced back from various setbacks. As you will see as you read on, there were plenty more challenges ahead.

CHAPTER 5

Never Lose Hope

There is no education like adversity.

DISRAELI

As the years rolled on, my life settled into a stable routine. I attended my annual follow-up appointments, and aside from ongoing issues with my wonky heart rhythm, everything seemed fine. I always knew that at some point I would be facing another valve replacement, but as technology moved on, I began to expect that this could be done through a catheter from a large vein in my groin, rather than having open-heart surgery.

The stress of opening my studio in 2012, running all the classes and taking care of everything – from the accounts, to the maintenance, to the administration – certainly took its toll. For a few years I almost lost track of 'me' and my goals in life. My desire to keep everyone happy and provide a great client experience meant that financially it was a disaster, but I never lost hope that I could make it a success.

In 2015, having somewhat neglected my own health and fitness, I re-joined the big chain gym where I had been a member while I was working at the hospital. I had missed the indoor cycling classes and the friends I had made there, and I knew that I needed a routine and someone to tell me what to do!

I am always looking for that elusive balance in all areas of my life. If I monitor my personal life, business life, health and relationships, all too often I can score highly in several areas to the detriment of others. Like many people, it is not until a disaster strikes that I realise how far off the track I have gone.

I am a self-motivated person, but I was having to work so hard to keep my life and business on track that I just wanted to have a stress-free time when I didn't have to plan my every move. I fell back into a routine that I enjoyed, attending regular classes, swimming for pleasure and running in the lanes around my house when the mood took me. I even started to entertain doing some races, but I was wary of the commitment that would take and how easily I tend to get carried away.

I have never been able to move beyond my competitive nature, and even now, only moderately fit compared with my highest levels, I thrived on pushing myself in everything I did. It was a rare class when I didn't experience distracting palpitations, where my heart rate seemed to take off all on its own regardless of my effort level. Although I had raised the issue several times with my doctors, the assumption had always been that these issues were benign.

Sadly, that turned out not to be the case, and after one Saturday morning cycle class in early February 2016, I followed my regular routine and went to the supermarket on the way home. While there, I noticed that I had a strange dark area in my vision at the bottom of my left eye. In retrospect, I should have gone straight to the eye hospital, but I didn't think it was anything serious. I didn't want to make a fuss or take time off work, and I thought it would just sort itself out, given time.

When I mentioned the issue to my friend Rachel several days later, she insisted that I needed to do something about it. I duly went along to the eye infirmary, saw a nurse and then a consultant. Nobody seemed to be too sure of a diagnosis, or whether the issue was related to a clot or swelling, but it was suggested that I should have a brain scan and be seen in the stroke clinic.

Unfortunately, that referral somehow got lost in the hospital system, and it wasn't until nearly three weeks later, after I had called to ask what had happened to my referral, that I got an urgent call to come in the next day. They were full of apologies for the 'administrative error', but by then the blackness had crept up and was completely covering the bottom half of my eye, leaving the top half blurry. On seeing the consultant, I was taken for a long-overdue brain scan.

I certainly didn't have any of the typical neurological symptoms of a stroke, but there wasn't any other simple explanation for my sight issues either. I was admitted to the acute stroke ward as a precaution while I waited for the results, and it was a surprised consultant who came to see me that evening. The scan showed not only that I had indeed had a recent optic nerve stroke, where the blood flow to my optic nerve had been blocked, but also that I had had a second 'historic' stroke, which was in the optical region of my brain.

Since nobody accurately knew when either of these events occurred, or if there was any underlying reason for what had happened, I was scheduled for a lumbar puncture the next day to rule out an inflammatory process or autoimmune disease, such as multiple sclerosis. What followed was one of the most sleep-deprived but funniest nights that I have ever spent in hospital.

Bed space was at a premium, and as I was under the care of the neurology team, I remained in a four-bed bay on the acute stroke ward. The other three occupants were in various states of dementia or post-stroke confusion. One was continually shouting out the name of her husband, Dennis, who had long since gone home when visiting hours were over. Another went through phases of repeatedly banging her water cup on the bedside cabinet to demand attention, while the third thought this was someone knocking on the door and responded by saying, 'Come in!'

The first few times it happened I could but laugh, but after it had been going on for hours it lost its amusement value. In the end, my only option was to go and get a few hours of sleep in the TV room, so I wasn't particularly rested come the next day. Thankfully, I was later moved to another area of the ward, where the occupants were younger, friendlier and not so unwell.

I waited most of the day for the lumbar puncture, which I will admit was one of the most painful and unpleasant procedures of my life. A junior doctor was assigned to get the required spinal fluid, and although he assured me that he had done so with success many times before, I lost count of the number of attempts he had to make. Each one involved several sub-cutaneous injections of local anaesthetic to numb the area, followed by poking a giant needle into the intervertebral disk spaces in my lower back.

No matter what he did, or the positions we tried, it just wasn't happening. I have a high pain tolerance, but I must admit that it was testing my good nature to the max and my language was becoming increasingly flowery as time went on. I strongly believe that everyone must learn, but after about six attempts we agreed that he should call his senior house officer for support.

The process started again with a lovely lady who, having ascertained that I had a slight spinal scoliosis (or an abnormal curvature) and that my disk spaces were particularly small, took a further three attempts before she eventually struck gold. To add to the humour of the situation, she had positioned me sitting on the side of the bed with my legs off the edge, leaning forward with my arms propped on the table in front of me. As the needle finally went in, it tweaked some nerves and my knee shot up and hit me in the eye socket. My leg continued to twitch madly as she excitedly asked me to stay still.

For the next week, I walked around looking like I had pooped in my trousers – not a good advertisement for someone who teaches exercise classes! The results would take several weeks to come through, and in the meantime I was put on a course of high-dose steroids to see if that would improve my vision.

I couldn't wait to get out of the hospital. Although it was suggested that I should stay at least another night, I insisted that I was going home later that evening and was discharged. Just as I had done after other traumatic events, I immersed myself into my work straight away and tried to carry on as if nothing had happened.

A couple of days later, I had a follow-up appointment at the eye infirmary. By now I had had several weeks to process the new reality of my situation, and I had experienced the gamut of emotions – from anger, to denial, to depression. My stroke was such an unexpected turn of events that it really caught me off balance. I had always imagined that I knew what my next trial would be, and it certainly wasn't to lose all my usable vision in one eye.

I had been playing games with myself to see if there was anything I could do to get quality sight back in my left eye. I tried everything, from walking around my house with a bandana over my good eye to see if I could train the bad one to get better, to sitting for ages in the hot tub at the gym with the idea that dilating my blood vessels might improve the flow. I spent hours on the internet trying to find somebody with my condition who had experienced an improvement, but most of what I learned indicated that around one-quarter of patients had the same thing happen to their other eye in a few years' time. That was a sobering thought, which led to a few tears.

I now know that optic nerve strokes mainly happen to elderly people with other significant health conditions, such as very high blood pressure or medicated low blood pressure, ischaemic heart disease, diabetes or rheumatoid arthritis. I had drawn the short straw, with valvular heart disease and some bad luck.

I was well prepared when I next saw the ophthalmologist. As he slowly pushed his chair back and away from the examination table, our eyes met. I could sense that he was taking his time to decide how best to relay his thoughts. Eventually he said, 'I am afraid that your optic nerve is very pale and ischaemic. I think it is unlikely that you will experience any improvement in your sight in that eye.' So that was it. No matter how strongly I willed it to happen or how often I tried to train my eye with silly exercises, it wasn't going to improve.

After a few moments of awkwardness, when I was convinced the poor doctor expected me to burst into tears, I simply nodded my head and smiled to defuse the tension. Although the fact that things were not going to improve at all was my worst-case scenario, it was the one I had already accepted as likely to come my way. I had held onto a little hope, but hearing his prognosis didn't come as much of a shock.

Kubler-Ross stages of grief model

This model was developed in 1969 by Swiss psychiatrist Elizabeth Kubler-Ross, following her work with terminally ill patients. She used it to describe the five emotional stages that someone facing a terminal diagnosis moves through: denial, anger, bargaining, depression and acceptance.

The author herself later noted that her fixed model didn't fit all situations and in reality people often experience these emotions in a different order and for varying periods of time. More recently, the model has been expanded into something called the change curve. This is a better way to help people understand their reactions to a major life-changing event, such as bereavement, divorce, redundancy, imprisonment or a critical health challenge.

As you read through this book, you will find examples of all those emotions. Where I disagree with change curve is that it suggests that there is an endpoint, and that once we reach acceptance we have fully come to terms with our new situation. It is acknowledged that we never really get over the loss of a loved one, and I believe this is also true for the grief that we feel when living with a long-term health condition.

What the model shows is that it is completely normal to experience these emotions when we are facing a life-changing situation. I used to question if feeling angry or depressed about what had happened meant that I was weak, but now I have a clear understanding that these negative emotions are a necessary part of the acceptance process. Providing we don't get stuck on one of the first four stages, there is always a way through. What acceptance looks like differs from person to person, so there is no clear prescription for achieving it.

I have also found that I can revisit certain emotions – often after a trigger, such as an ill-thought-through comment by a friend or a hospital appointment arriving in the post. The positive thing about this for me is that having processed these emotions before, it seems to be easier to get through them again.

The loss of sight was a new experience for me. Throughout my other medical challenges, I had always believed that I could work hard to overcome my limitations. Yet no amount of training was going to bring my left eye back, and I would be stuck with the very limited amount of vision I had in it for ever. While I can sometimes go for hours or even days without being reminded of the restrictions caused by my heart, I am constantly reminded that I no longer have biopic vision.

Nothing – from reading to driving, from opening a door to accurately judging distance – is as easy as it was. The little things annoy me the most. Shut your left eye and try wiping deodorant on your armpit or pinning a clothes peg on the washing line, and you will understand some of the daily irritations I face caused by limited perception of depth.

Most worrying of all was the thought that I could lose my driver's licence. I surrendered it to the DVLA as soon as my problem set in, and I didn't get it back until after they had sent me for an official eye test to prove that the vision in my right eye met the required standard and that I still had a good enough visual field. I had prepared myself for the worst case, so keeping my licence was a happy bonus.

I still grieve for the sight I have lost. It's the one thing I would change in my life if I could. I am eternally grateful that neither of my strokes caused significant neurological damage, but they were a great reminder that life can change in the blink of an eye – pun intended!

What I have fortunately never lost throughout my journey is a feeling of hope. Even in my darkest moments, I had a belief that things could and would get better. The American psychologist Charles Snyder theorised that hope is a cognitive skill that enables us to maintain our focus in the pursuit of a goal. He reasoned that our ability to remain hopeful in the face of obstacles depended on two types of thinking: pathway thinking and agency thinking.

Agency thinking refers to our belief that we have the power to instigate change to help ourselves reach our goals, whereas pathway thinking relates to our capacity to consider different options for how we could do so. For anyone in my position it can be particularly hard to maintain hope when we have so little control over our future health. My way of dealing with that uncertainty has been to attach my sense of optimism to the things that I can do to influence my outcomes, rather than to achieving what I view as optimal health.

Although I have always maintained a belief in my ability to recover from various setbacks, I have also been forced to accept that things outside my control may affect the completeness of any recovery. As much as I always hope that I will be unfettered by my health history, I try to ensure that my positivity and identity are not based entirely on the achievement of a predetermined health outcome.

As I see it, no matter how bad things get, I can always make things better than they are today. In times of medical challenge, I have centred my goals around things that I can control, such as eating well or still getting regular exercise – things that I hope will affect my outcome rather than the outcome itself. In my mind, when I lose hope, then my illness has won.

CHAPTER 6

Look For The Positives
In Your Adversity

An arrow can only be shot by pulling it backward. When life is dragging you back with difficulties, it means it's going to launch you into something great. So just focus, and keep aiming.

UNKNOWN AUTHOR

It is perhaps unsurprising that I struggled mentally with losing my vision. Over the years I had learned to cope with challenges to my sense of self, but I had now lost a lot of confidence in my body. After all the things that had happened to me, I felt I didn't deserve to have been presented with this additional obstacle.

Realistically, I know that the course of life isn't about what you do or don't deserve. Bad things just happen, and the only real recourse is to deal with them and move forward. That said, it was so unexpected that for a while I found myself stuck in something of a negative rut, asking 'why me?'

Since nobody could succinctly tell me what had happened or why, I became fearful that the same thing could happen in my other eye and that I would be left effectively blind. I started playing out scenarios in my head and dwelling on what would happen if they became a reality. I found myself waking up at night and being unable to get back to sleep. I felt overly anxious every time I had a little twitch in my good eye or my heart rhythm acted up. The trouble was, the more I dwelt on it, the bigger my fear and feelings of impending doom became.

In my early twenties, I listened to a motivational tape (yes, it was that long ago), where the word fear was used as an acronym for False Evidence Appearing Real. Although not all my evidence was false, it certainly grew out of control and started to dominate my thoughts. In the end, I realised that I had to take back control of my mindset, and the easiest way to do this was to confront my biggest fear and weaken its power.

I actively sought out online videos and documentaries about people with vision impairments, especially those who had managed to maintain an active lifestyle. I was particularly inspired by the visually impaired para-triathletes, who managed to swim and run with a fully sighted guide and do the cycle portion of the race on a tandem. I found comfort in the fact that even if I did become blind in the future, I would still be able to live a full and active life. That realisation took a lot of the fear away.

I also acknowledged that I needed to be much kinder to myself, and to be more forgiving of and open about my shortcomings. I had always wanted to be perceived as invincible and mentally strong, yet this challenge had led to a real emotional blip. My belief had always been that expressing any form of vulnerability was a weakness, and that the solution was to pull on some 'big girl pants' and get on with it.

I preferred to hide my inner struggles and show a tough exterior to the world. In doing so, I had shut out a lot of people who could have helped me. That aloofness has been not only a strength, but a weakness. The battle to allow others fully into my life is one I am still fighting. I am fully aware that it is rather hypocritical to see it as my mission to help others on their own journey if I am not prepared to accept that support in return.

I wouldn't be human if I didn't experience some fear and doubt about my future health. I think that living with a long-term illness is particularly hard, and often more so mentally than physically.

The theory is that you learn to deal with that situation by integrating the new you with the old you, keeping the parts of your identity that are congruent and shedding those that are not. With long-term illness, all too often aspects of the trauma continue into the present. There can be constant daily reminders in the form of medications, scars, physical limitations, symptoms worsening or recurring, and the very real fear that it is when, and not if, we will get ill again.

I have needed to not only incorporate my experiences and current reality into my plans, but also to have at least a passing awareness of potential risk. We all must deal with uncertainty in our lives, and a medical emergency can happen to anyone out of the blue. Living with a long-term health condition adds a layer of complication to many aspects of everyday existence. Although I am determined not to let it stop me pursuing my hopes and dreams, I would be lying if I didn't admit that it has an impact.

Even something as simple as taking a holiday, especially overseas, involves ensuring that I have enough medication, taking out specialist and often expensive travel insurance, being at least a little aware of where the big cardiac hospitals are in case of an emergency, making sure that somebody with me knows a little of my history should I be taken ill, and accepting that I shouldn't visit remote places where rudimental care could not be quickly found.

I have, of course, ignored all my self-imposed rules over the years; I have travelled without insurance, to remote places, on my own. Breaking those logical rules is, I suppose, a way of asserting my independence. It also says something about my attitude to risk versus reward, which has changed at different points in my life. We all must decide where we lie on that spectrum, and I am in the somewhat privileged position of having no dependents. If there were children, a husband or a significant other involved, I would have to think about someone other than myself.

Dealing with uncertainty

One of the more difficult aspects of living with a long-term health condition is coping with uncertainty. Everything from waiting for hospital test results to fearing getting ill again can gnaw away at our ability to enjoy the present moment – if we let it.

1. Don't catastrophise. When facing uncertainty, it's easy to dwell on the worst-case scenario, rather than maintain optimism and balance. Unfortunately, worrying unnecessarily about things before they happen, especially scenarios that may never happen, sucks us into a dark place. Worrying doesn't usually change the outcome, but it makes us less able to stay positive.

2. Decide which factors you can control and which you can't. When waiting for hospital tests or results, for instance, how long they take is generally out of our control. Being annoyed about delays will only drain our energy.

3. Focus on the present. Most of us project our fears into the future and worry about things that haven't happened yet. If

we instead choose to be truly present and celebrate the here and now, it's easier to take back control of our emotions.

4. Find a positive in every scenario. We tend to focus on the negative possibilities, but what if even those had an upside? When I couldn't stop dwelling on the possibility of fully losing my sight, I decided to embrace that fear. In doing so, I took away its power to dominate my thoughts.

5. Take some form of positive action. Uncertainty can paralyse us and prevent us from doing anything. Instead, begin a new project, go for a walk, enjoy some music or talk things through with a close friend.

6. Know that you will cope, whatever the outcome. If the worst does happen, be confident that you will be able to find a way to deal with it.

I have always anticipated that I won't make old bones, and as I age my quality of life is likely to be increasingly affected by my condition. I don't see that as a terrible thing, as it encourages me to live for today, and not dwell on the past or look too far into the future. What I don't want to do is to lead my life in a bubble. I don't want to allow those 'what ifs' to take away my quest to push my boundaries and get the most out of every day.

I can't easily control what happens to me, but I always have a choice in how to react. Knowing I have that choice has been one of the biggest positives for my mental health. Often, if I speak with someone who is really struggling with an obstacle in life, they have failed to see that they still have control over how they perceive their situation. I'm not saying that we should be falsely happy about bad things, but if we only see the negative or seek to blame somebody or something else for the cards that life deals us, that is a route to misery and resentment. I have 100 per cent responsibility for the quality of my thoughts.

If we listen to our internal dialogue, often its comments are negative. I dare you to tune in and really assess how you talk to yourself. We berate ourselves for our weaknesses, dwell on our failures, call ourselves names and invent a myriad of excuses for why our life doesn't look how we think it should. Part of that is an evolutionary response designed to help us assess risk and stay safe, but often those negative thoughts can prevent us from finding a constructive way forward.

I have taught myself strategies to deal with my negative thoughts, so I don't let them consume me. Much as I might have a 'head in the sand' personality, I am self-aware enough to know that sooner or later I must deal with my emotions and confront my fears. Although this process is uncomfortable at times, it is the only way to reduce their power and hold.

I have a series of questions that I like to ask myself:

- Is this a realistic fear?
- Is there good evidence that it could happen?
- Is there anything I can do to reduce the chance of it coming true?
- Is there an alternative way of framing it, where I could find a positive?
- What could I do to find benefit, even if the worst happened?

The final question is particularly important to me, because once I have worked through what I would do if the fear became a reality, I have much less reason to be scared. Although it might sound strange, my biggest fear is never death. I do not fear dying, but having to live with a significant disability that takes away my ability to lead a reasonably full and active life.

It happens to everyone in the end. As we age, our physical capabilities diminish and we are forced to accept that fewer life options are on the table. Yet I look at some of my clients, several of whom are in their late eighties, and I realise that they are still leading full and active lives. Their options may be fewer, but they are making the most of the capability they still have.

Life can be unpredictable when it comes to living with a long-term health condition. Physical or mental capability can be taken away sooner than expected, and rather than there being a gradual decline the situation can change overnight. There is little point in spending too much time mourning what you have lost, as the focus needs to be on looking after what you still have.

I have often struggled with whether to label myself as having a disability, so I have tended to avoid it. The word conjures up an expectation of losing a facet of life that is considered normal, and sadly society can be harsh in its judgement. For me, there is a dichotomy between the desire to maintain my independence and the acknowledgement that in the future I may well need extra help.

My sense of self and my identity are so intrinsically linked to my ability to express myself physically that completely losing that ability would make it hard for me to carry on. I fought extremely hard to rebuild myself after my second open-heart surgery, and I applied the same methodology after the stroke. My physical fitness wasn't immediately changed by the loss of vision, but my ability to enjoy the activities that I considered part of my identity certainly was.

Perhaps saddest of all was that I completely lost confidence that I would ever ride my beloved bike again. Cycling classes in the gym were a substitute, but nothing could totally replace the buzz I got from riding outside. The amount of road cycling I did had markedly reduced since I returned from Florida, but I still loved the freedom of taking myself away from my house and onto the moors, or even just a few miles to the local shop.

Riding a bike is not like being in a car. There you are protected from dodgy road surfaces and potholes, you keep a safe distance from other road users, and the consequences of a miscalculation usually only mean a dab on the brakes or a press on the accelerator. When cycling, you rely on all your senses to work together. When in a group, you want to ride close to each other not only because it makes conversation easier but also because it is more efficient, as you shield each other from the wind. Although the sight in my good eye needed no correction, I had lost much of my depth perception, clarity and fine judgement of distance. The peripheral vision on my left is non-existent unless I move my head, and, of course, it is impossible to look forward and sideways at the same time while riding. I thought that my cycling days were done and fell into a bit of a funk.

Yet again, some friends came to my rescue. Two amazing buddies, both called Mike, whom I had been going to indoor cycle classes with for years, kept encouraging me to join them on their weekend group rides. I was resistant at first, but I eventually decided to confront my fears head-on.

One quiet Sunday morning, we all met up at the gym and did a lovely 26-mile route out to Dartmoor and back. The Mikes were great at making sure I was OK, and little by little, over several weeks, my confidence began to return. We were joined by Julie, and she and I struck up a great friendship. We rode most weekends together, even through the depths of the winter.

I know that I am never going to be the calibre of cyclist I was when I was at my racing peak, before my surgeries and the loss of sight in my left eye, but I am unbelievably happy that my passion for cycling has not been taken away entirely. Equally, without the encouragement of the Mikes and Julie, I may never have found the courage to try. For that I will always be grateful.

As much as I felt the need to resume all aspects of my old life to prove that I was unchanged by what had happened, I also recognised that if I wanted to fully accept my new situation, I had to stop clinging desperately to the person I was before. I found that process extremely difficult. My heart condition had always been easy to hide if I wanted to, but my sight issues were not so simple to disguise. My coping strategy was to deliberately put myself in situations where people only knew me as someone with a visual impairment.

That new challenge inevitably came in the form of a physical activity, in this case kayaking. I had only basic skills so there was huge room for improvement, and it didn't require vast amounts of physical strength or fitness. It was also sociable, so I could make new friends, and coaching and support were available at a local club.

The members of the Port of Plymouth Canoe and Kayak Association were incredibly welcoming and endlessly encouraging despite my evident lack of skill. I didn't try to hide my sight issues, and paddling near others made me uncomfortable to begin with. I was forever bumping into other boats, especially if they appeared unexpectedly on my left-hand side. I learned to make fun of my situation, and as my ability to control speed and direction improved, I had to apologise less.

It would have been easy to stay in my comfort zone, with people who already knew me, and to avoid putting myself in situations where this new disability had an impact. But then I knew that my life would get smaller, and where would that end? I would build up a whole load of reasons not to do things, some real and some perceived, and I felt sure that the list would grow if I let it.

Another key to maintaining my sense of optimism is to actively seek the benefits in whatever situation I find myself in. When faced with a life-changing event or trauma, it's easy to become focused on the negatives of the situation. I had little trouble finding the benefits in my 2005 heart surgery, but I really struggled when it came to my stroke. For a long time, all I could understand was what I had lost.

Eventually I realised that I had gained a heightened sense of empathy for others and how they deal with their struggles. I have learned so much from the amazing people I have met. Sometimes I can forget that other people have not yet had the opportunity to develop higher levels of inner strength, or that their story is filled with much greater adversity than mine, which can take longer to process. Providing I always do my best to support the people in my life as best as I can, I am fulfilling my own remit.

Given my own brushes with depression, self-loathing and the abandonment of responsibility, I wish that I didn't find it so hard to be around people who are stuck in that mindset. I like to think that I am understanding, but my protective mechanism seems to be to distance myself from people who are permanently locked in that battle. Occasional wobbles are part of life, and my only prerequisite for wanting to help people is that they express a desire to be better. Feeling down is fine, but deciding that things can never improve is not. My best learning experiences have come from being forced to overcome hardship, rather than from doing things that go completely to plan. Far from diminishing my life and what I have achieved, facing obstacles has added to it.

I have never viewed myself as a particularly resilient person, but I have always found ways to move forward after setbacks. I certainly don't want to waste precious time by feeling sorry for myself or thinking that life owes me something because of what has happened. With each successive life obstacle, I have had to assimilate many changes. I have become more adept at fighting to maintain certain aspects of my life while filling those parts irretrievably lost with other rewards. Rather as in Professor Stephen Joseph's shattered vase theory, mentioned in Chapter 1, I have been able to take the many fragments of my life and rebuild them into what I consider to be a rather fine mural!

I don't judge how others choose to deal with their own hardship, but for me, allowing adversity to define who I am and what I do with the rest of my life would mean missing out on so many wonderful opportunities and experiences. We only come this way once, or, depending on our belief system, we could come back as a slimy slug. It is important to live without regret.

Hardship has also taught me that I can be strong. Rather like the time in hospital when I couldn't reach my breakfast bowl, we are all at some point faced with a choice. I know I am not here to be a victim of my circumstances. I can win in life because I choose to see these potential negatives as assets, not things that hold me back.

6. Look For The Positives In Your Adversity

Resilience is like a muscle that can be trained. Far from beating us down, consistent challenges can build us up and give us more capacity to face the next adversity. And come our way that will. Our level of resilience defines the resources we can draw on when facing adversity. Little did I know when I had my stroke just how much I would have to draw on those reserves only a year later.

CHAPTER 7

You Are Stronger Than You Think

We have no right to ask when sorrow comes, 'Why did this happen to me?' unless we ask the same question for every moment of happiness that comes our way.

UNKNOWN AUTHOR

Life again settled into something of a routine after the stroke. I made some significant improvements in my work-life balance by consolidating my business and closing one of the two studios I had at that point. With a little extra free time, I could focus on getting fitter. I was in the gym three or four times each week, swimming, cycling or running. As much as the weather allowed, I was out on my bike with Julie on a Sunday morning. My confidence returned to the point that I re-joined the local running club after a hiatus of about five years, and I went out on group runs a couple of times each week.

I certainly wasn't fast, or anywhere near the standard I used to be, but having a slightly more relaxed attitude enabled me to get enjoyment from what I could still achieve. At the back of my mind,

I wanted to set myself a big goal to work towards, and in late October I committed to race in Ironman UK the following August.

Ironman was unfinished business for me, having failed at my one attempt way back in 2001, when I was at the peak of my fitness and ability. To successfully race an Ironman distance triathlon, with its 2.4-mile swim, 112-mile bike ride and 26.2-mile run, takes large volumes of training in all three sports, a good plan and a bit of luck. I had put together a great season of racing, and I was on track to achieve my eleven-hour time goal, when on my way back from the local pool I was knocked off my bike by a hotel valet. I was incredibly fortunate not to be seriously injured, but with a bunch of road rash and extensive bruising I lost a few weeks of key training just a month before my big race.

Hindsight is a wonderful thing, but I made a huge training mistake when I allowed my fear of failure to dominate my normally pragmatic mind. Ironman was the pinnacle of my athletic goals at that point, and I panicked when I felt that my ability to have an exceptional race was in jeopardy. I have always been a notorious over-trainer, impatient with my body and fitness and perhaps too willing to regularly dig into my reserves rather than rest.

I recognise that this stems from my childhood and my desire to live a life without excuses, without giving others any leeway in their expectations of my physical ability. I suppose that is why I had been so drawn to long-distance triathlon in the first place, with its association with high-achiever, type-A personalities who are willing to push themselves beyond the norm.

Triathlon is also a highly individual sport, so I could never find myself as the weakest link in a team. In my school days, I was often one of the last to be chosen in any team physical activity. That feeling of being viewed as inferior had left its mark. In triathlon, I only had to rely on my ability to make the most of my potential. It appealed to my perfectionist nature – no matter how good I was, I always thought I could be better.

After the bike accident, instead of reducing my training to give my body time to be fully rested by race day, I caught up on the key long sessions I thought I had missed. On the long drive from south Florida to Pensacola Beach a day before the race, I knew I was in trouble. Instead of feeling excited and filled with energy, I was, in athletic terms, flat. My get up and go had got up and gone – not the situation you want to be in ahead of a long and gruelling day.

The next morning, even before the gun went, I was despondent. My eleven-hour race plan was looking more like twelve or thirteen, and the thought of toiling so far beneath what I believed to be my true potential filled me with dread. I don't live with regrets, but I made one of the few decisions in life that I wish I could undo. As the gun went, I walked into the sea and began the first of two laps. The further I swam, the worse I felt. Endurance athletics is as much a mental as a physical game, and in my mind I was already beaten. As I finally hit the beach, ready to run around the flags and back out on the second lap, I did something I have never done before or since. I gave up.

Just like that, I sat down and cried. I was angry with myself for making such a rookie training mistake and pushing on when I should have been backing off. I blamed the valet for leaving me in this position, when in fact my own poor decision making had been as much at fault as theirs. While my friends all went on to have reasonable races, I looked for excuses and returned to my hotel room mentally broken.

Looking back, I should have faced up to my own poor choices and slogged on that day. It wouldn't have been pretty, and I would have been out there a lot longer than I had hoped, but I would have salvaged something and not been left feeling like a complete failure. The irony is that I was at the peak of my fitness – these days, there is no chance of me having a twelve, thirteen or even fifteen-hour race!

It took me several weeks to process what had happened, to stop blaming the valet parker and come to terms with how I had sabotaged my own race. Every cloud has a silver lining, and mine was that I went on to use my super-high fitness levels to do a brilliant half-ironman race. I spent the next six months setting personal records at every running, cycling and triathlon event I attended.

I entered countless running and cycling races in the intervening years, but still the Ironman failure grated on me. There was an element of redemption in mind when, fifteen years later in October 2016, I pressed the online entry button. Yet again, unfortunately, I would discover that life had other ideas.

By early 2017 I had put together a solid winter of training, and everything was going to plan. I was far from the athlete I had once been, and my heart health was certainly holding me back. I was getting increasingly breathless when running or cycling uphill, but I still felt confident that I could improve my fitness and have a decent race.

In late February, I came home after a Saturday morning cycle class at the gym and started to feel unwell. I was hot, cold and feeling sick. Thinking that I had a stomach bug, I went to bed, but I began to feel increasingly rough. I was either shivering so much that my teeth rattled together or pouring in sweat, which soaked the bed sheets. Over the next few days I couldn't stray far from my bed. I was retching even though I hadn't eaten anything, and I was becoming increasingly dysfunctional. I decided to call NHS 111 for advice.

I explained my predicament, but somehow in their line of questioning I had answered 'yes' to a question about whether I was having heart palpitations. I certainly was, and they were worse than usual, probably because I had a shocking fever. I didn't see it as my main issue, but it turned out to be one of their 'red flag' questions. Despite my protests, I couldn't convince them that I didn't need an ambulance.

The paramedics turned up and I let them into the house while apologising for wasting their time. One of them was a keen cyclist and we spent some time discussing the merits of the four bikes that were cluttering up my tiny cottage. They took a basic patient history and then insisted that I go to the ambulance for an echocardiogram (ECG) or heart trace, and to allow them to fully examine me. They concluded that my symptoms suggested I had some form of infection. I had vowed after a bad experience before my 2005 surgery that the only way I was going back to A&E was when I had no choice and was on a gurney. Sensing this, they told me I should go to my GP the next morning.

I wasn't capable of driving, so my loyal friend Mark took me. I must have looked a bit of a sight, as it didn't take the GP long to diagnose pyelonephritis, a kidney infection. He wanted me to go to hospital, but he agreed that if I could keep down some high-dose antibiotics and if I started to feel better within twelve hours, I could avoid it. Thankfully, that was what happened. A kidney scan a week later showed nothing unusual, and I thought the episode was over.

The second issue reared its head just as that one was getting sorted out. After my stroke, having to take more blood thinners had left me with significant bleeding issues during my period. Investigations had shown that I had a large fibroid (a benign tumour), which wasn't helping the situation. The heavy bleeding had made me very anaemic, so with a referral from my cardiologist I had a coil put in, which stopped the monthly bleeding for about seven months.

Then, suddenly, at the same time as the kidney infection, I started bleeding heavily. A week later, the coil washed out. I tried to get an urgent appointment with a gynaecologist, but they told me I had been signed off and that my only option was to go to my GP and ask them to put it back in. Without a female doctor on staff, they referred me on. After waiting a week to get an appointment at a local clinic, I was again told that due to my medical history they couldn't help me.

I was at my wits' end, with the bleeding so bad that no sanitary protection would deal with it, and I was getting increasingly weak. My house looked like a murder scene, with blood all over the furniture, floor and bed sheets. Things came to a head a few days later, when after a particularly torrid night, when I had barely slept, I was feeling terribly dizzy and having trouble standing up. Fearing for my safety, at around 6am I had little choice but to call an ambulance.

This time I was willing let them escort me to Derriford Hospital, as I didn't know what else to do. My blood pressure was low and getting lower, and even the two paramedics looked concerned. I was wheeled into a side room, where I was mortified to soak the sheets. A little blood goes an awfully long way!

An A&E doctor took my history and went off to consult her colleagues. It so happened that the standard medication to stop the bleeding quickly, tranexamic acid, was completely out of the question for someone with a history of stroke. With the doctor not being entirely sure how to proceed, I was sent to the gynaecology ward to wait for a specialist.

The only workable solution was norethisterone, a progesterone pill, but it would take several days to stem the flow. I also got an appointment for a few weeks later, on Tuesday 28 March, to have the coil put back in. I thought this might be the end of the saga, but unfortunately it was just the beginning.

Once the bleeding stopped I was hopeful that I would start to feel better, but instead things got worse. The A&E admission showed that I was very anaemic, so I was prescribed iron tablets. I was struggling to function at all, just about making it into work each day but then barely able to climb the stairs to my studio. I was incapable of doing anything but sitting in my office chair and teaching by wheeling myself around the room.

By the end of the day I could just about make it home to my cottage before collapsing on the sofa, where I would spend the rest of the evening. Going upstairs to the bathroom or to bed was a trial, and more than once I passed out before I got there. I resorted to crawling, as it seemed to be the safest option. I took to buying microwave meals on the way home, but even this stopped when I had a panic in the store one night and realised I was going to pass out before I made it to the till.

My heart rate, normally in the low fifties at rest, rarely fell below 100. Exhausted as I was, I could barely sleep at night because of the sound of rushing blood in my ears. It wouldn't have taken a genius to realise that I was very unwell, but concluding that I was simply anaemic, I continued to wait for the gynaecology appointment. I went to Derriford on Tuesday 28 March, parked, and very slowly made my way to gynaecology. By then, all I could do was sit and flop against a wall, and I was relieved when I was taken to an examination room and invited to lie on the bed.

Several doctors and hours later, a coil was found and put in. I was advised to stay on the norethisterone for another two weeks until the progesterone from the coil had built up enough to stop me bleeding again. Blood tests also showed that my haemoglobin levels, or iron levels, were dramatically low. Sensing how unwell I was, the doctor advised me to wait until I could have a unit of blood to try and restore my levels.

It finally arrived from the blood bank late in the afternoon, but just before setting up the two-hour infusion, a nurse took my temperature and noted that it was raised. That meant I could no longer have the blood, as it would be impossible to tell if I was having a bad reaction if I already had a fever. Frustratingly, I was sent away with the proviso that I should come back a few days later to try again.

By then it was early evening. I walked out of the hospital into the dark and the pouring rain and tried to get to my car, which was parked some distance away. I just wanted to go home and sleep, but looking back I should really have insisted that I stay. I blacked out three times on the way to my car, and even when I got there I was forced to lie down by the passenger door, soaked to the skin. Eventually I got inside, and after a short nap I felt OK to drive home.

I have never been one to shirk responsibility, so the next day, as usual, I went to work. Over the preceding few weeks my lovely clients had been getting increasingly concerned, but I kept assuring them that everything was in hand and that I would be all right. I couldn't stand that feeling of vulnerability, so I employed my usual tactic of carrying on regardless.

Two days later, when I could eventually make it out of bed, I went back to Derriford Hospital, this time with the hope that I would get the much-needed unit of blood. Again, I spent several hours sitting in the waiting room while it was brought up from the blood bank, but this time a nurse had checked that my temperature was all right before ordering it.

I wasn't thinking clearly and my mobile was on silent, but eventually I noticed that my phone had rung. I went outside to return the call, and it was a message from the cardiology department upstairs asking me to get in touch urgently. I went back into the ward to collect my bag so I could go upstairs to speak to them, and the gynaecology doctor stopped me to say that she had heard from cardiology too. The blood they had taken on Tuesday had shown that I had a serious infection, most probably growing in my prosthetic heart valve, and I needed urgent medical treatment.

Bizarrely, because I wasn't an inpatient, I couldn't be transferred between departments. Instead, they told me to go out of the main hospital, go around the corner to A&E, admit myself and sit there until they came to find me.

Boosting your inner strength

Inner strength is something you perhaps don't know you have until you really need it. Having worked with people dealing with all sorts of medical challenges over the years, I find it interesting that some people seem to be emotionally weakened by what is happening, yet others gain in strength. It is inevitable that we all have moments of self-doubt and anxiety, and it isn't always easy to maintain positivity and optimism.

I have always viewed my inner strength like a muscle, in that continually nurturing it increases its ability to work in my favour when it needs to. In a way, it is why I don't fear the onset of further adversity. We will all have to face significant difficulties at some point in our lives, be it medical, financial or emotional, so I choose to see those challenges as a way for me to hone my strength. The harder or more frequent the fight, the more I can grow.

I suppose the only danger from this approach would be if I ended up feeling invincible, or became inflexible in my ability to adapt. Rather like the Japanese proverb 'The bamboo that bends is stronger than the oak that resists', my self-belief that I can always accept both the good and the bad in any situation has stood me in good stead.

I have several techniques I like to use when my inner strength is wavering:

- I remind myself that I have survived before and will again
- I make plans for the future, beyond the current crisis
- I share my struggles with friends and family, who I know will support me
- I make time to exercise – nurturing my physical strength translates into mental strength
- I give back, taking the focus away from me and direct it onto other people
- I seek positive achievements every day by doing things that I know I can achieve
- I document my journey, so I can look back later and see how far I have come
- I trust my instincts and believe in myself

People often comment on my inner strength and positivity, and my most frequent reply is 'What's the alternative?' To me, giving up is not an option. Withering away, feeling sorry for myself, or failing to maximise my potential would seem like a waste of the gift of life I have been given and the time I have left. Thinking about my death may not be comfortable, but it acts as a constant reminder to make the most of opportunities while I am here.

I also believe that my ability to adapt and overcome is not exceptional. Everyone has that skill within them if they are prepared to let it shine. The more life beats you down, the greater your opportunity to thrive. Challenges may change you, but they only take away your strength if you let them.

CHAPTER 8

Relish The Challenge

Bad is never good until worse happens.

DANISH PROVERB

I struggled to follow even those basic instructions and it took me a long time to make my way to A&E without falling over. My mind was in overdrive. As a congenital heart patient with a valve replacement, I have always known that I was at risk of getting endocarditis, an infection in the lining of the heart and its valves. The second that endocarditis was mentioned, I knew that their diagnosis was right. I felt such an idiot for not having figured it out myself in the weeks before. Foolishly, I had been holding on to the belief that anaemia was my only problem, and that had blinded me to any other possibility.

I had attributed the symptoms of endocarditis – extreme fatigue, night sweats and breathlessness – to anaemia. At one point, the amazing congenital heart specialist nurse in Plymouth, had asked me in an email if I thought I should get blood-culture tests done to rule endocarditis out, but I had dismissed the idea. It was not one of my finer moments, and that belief in my own invincibility could have cost me my life.

A little team from cardiology came and found me sitting sheepishly in A&E. Taking me to a side room, they explained that the tests showed I was harbouring an infection of staphylococcus lugdunensis, a highly aggressive bacterium. It was most likely now festering away and eating up my pulmonary valve, and to save my life I was going to be admitted to the hospital for at least six weeks of intravenous antibiotics. It was also likely that I would need another open-heart surgery to repair the damage.

Even when confronted with the evidence, I felt resistant, assuring them that hospitalisation was not an option. After all, I had a business to run. I was strongly advised not to leave the hospital, but I assured them that I needed to get my car out of the car park, go home, make some phone calls and pay some bills, and that I would return a few hours later. It is laughable that my mind instantly went into 'disaster mitigation and control' mode, even when presented with compelling evidence. I am not sure that I fully appreciated the gravity of my situation.

I did as I promised, and a few hours later I returned to the hospital, admitted myself to the ward and was taken for an echocardiogram to confirm the diagnosis. Sure enough, my heart was massively enlarged. Not only was my pulmonary valve almost blocked by vegetation and swelling, meaning my heart was struggling to pump against the resistance, but there was also a nasty abscess. The other valve on the right-hand side of my heart, the tricuspid, was also dramatically leaking due to the increased pressure. It wasn't a pretty picture.

The next day, aside from some units of blood to help with the anaemia, I had a CT scan to rule out a pulmonary embolism (a blood clot in the lung). All my records were sent to the congenital heart specialist unit in Bristol for review and a treatment plan. It was decided that I needed to be transferred urgently to the Bristol Heart Institute, and thus began one of the more amusing parts of this mess.

Two wonderful male paramedics were charged with getting me there, and I was duly packaged up on a gurney and rolled into the ambulance. We set off with flashing blues, ostensibly because they didn't want to get delayed in the rush-hour traffic. We chatted a lot, making light of my evident predicament in an attempt to defuse some of the tension. I would be lying if I said I wasn't worried, but because I had figured out that I had to surrender myself to whatever was going to happen in the coming weeks, my anxiety was surprisingly low.

It was now dark, and I couldn't see much from my prone position in the back of the ambulance other than glimpses through the window. It turned out that neither the driver nor the co-pilot in the back with me was sure where they were going, but thankfully the GPS kept us roughly on track. The route it chose was in over the Bristol suspension bridge. Unfortunately, having never been that way before, the driver failed to slow down enough as we hit the first speed bump at the entry to the bridge.

Everything took to the air, and we landed with a resounding bang. There was a lot of shouting, and having just about retrieved our brains from the top of our skulls, we slowed down just enough before hitting the exit bump. Having ascertained that I was OK, I joked that they had better not hold me responsible for any damage to the ambulance. The co-pilot commented that it wasn't his responsibility either, as it was his last day with the ambulance service. We all laughed.

I am familiar with the layout of the old Bristol Royal Infirmary and the children's hospital next to it, but not so much with the Bristol Heart Institute, a newer building opened in 2009 and shoehorned into the back of the site. The paramedics, similarly unsure, saw a sign that looked appropriate as we approached the children's hospital (I could see the recognisable coloured rings through the window) and turned in. What followed was a lot of banging on the roof as we went under the restricted height sign, followed by a similar noise as the ambulance reversed the other way, coupled with a second dose of good-humoured shouting.

They eventually found a suitable place to park the ambulance a little further on, and with some helpful directions through the rabbit warren of corridors, we arrived at the coronary care unit, which looked to be my designated stop for the next few days. After an uneventful handover I was quite sorry to see them go, suddenly feeling lonely and uncertain.

I didn't like being on the coronary care unit, and several of the nurses commented that it was a strange place for me to be, because I didn't have acquired heart disease. Worst of all, although I had a private room it had no windows, except some covered by a blind and facing the centre of the ward. I was attached to some basic monitoring equipment, so the furthest I could get was from the bed to the bathroom without setting off all sorts of alarms. The isolation and lack of contact bothered me, probably because it left me too much alone with my thoughts, with little distraction to quell the internal dialogue.

Over the weekend I had a minor procedure to put a peripherally inserted central catheter (PICC) into the brachial vein on the inside of my arm, with the tip threaded to reach the top of my heart. The PICC line was a godsend, as I knew that I was going to need many weeks of intravenous antibiotics. Although I am not bothered by needles, this permanent device saved a lot of hassle.

My blood results continued to show that I was still terribly anaemic, so I received another two units of blood to try to correct the situation. My antibiotics were 'pushed' into the PICC line four times each day: a half-hour infusion at 6am, 12pm, 6pm and 12am. Being a person who thrives on routine, I liked the organised nature of a hospital. Once I aligned my habits with theirs, things became simple.

In my little panicked trip home before being admitted to Derriford, I had thought to pack my iPad, so I was able to contact my friends. Rachel, my most wonderful buddy from my days working at the hospital, stayed in regular text contact, which always cheered me up. Mum made the train journey up and back several times, and, realising how dire the situation was, Mark cut short his overseas business trip to visit me. A lovely friend of mine, Nigel, whom I had first met in 2006 when I was doing my personal trainer course in Bristol, also dropped by, along with Caroline, a fellow congenital heart patient who lived locally. I certainly wasn't lacking in support from near or far.

My mind was still struggling to process how I had got into this mess. I wondered if I could have prevented it happening had I recognised earlier that I had endocarditis symptoms rather than just anaemia. Had my tendency to bury my head in the sand when confronted with medical issues contributed to my situation? Ultimately, I concluded that the how and why really didn't matter, as I couldn't take back my decisions. The only focus now needed to be on what I could do to get better.

The congenital heart team stopped by the next Monday morning, and that gave me a much-needed understanding of how they expected things to progress. I have always been able to deal with all sorts of challenges, but I find uncertainty difficult. I was much happier once I knew the plan was for me to receive several weeks of antibiotics to reduce my infection levels, then have surgery to replace my pulmonary valve and probably repair the tricuspid, and then another load of antibiotics until I was clear of the infection. An echocardiogram (often shortened to echo) was scheduled for the next day, and I settled in, expecting to follow their treatment plan.

The next afternoon in the echo suite, I was unusually quiet. Unlike in Derriford Hospital, where I know many of the technicians and often talk with them about their work, here I felt rather alone and only formal interactions took place. The porter had barely finished wheeling me back into my room when I saw a new man I didn't recognise standing in the doorway. When he introduced himself as the surgeon for congenital heart conditions, I realised how quickly things were accelerating out of my control.

He was holding the dreaded pink consent forms, and quickly explained that the results of my scan were more worrying than expected. He said that my heart was struggling. He had, as he put it, 'ordered the necessary parts', and I was scheduled for urgent surgery first thing on Thursday morning. I instantly liked him, as I have always preferred a direct approach over sugar-coating. Years of reading research papers to understand my own condition, and indeed congenital heart defects in general, have made me a reasonably well-educated patient. Nothing makes me more concerned than an apparent withholding of information.

Having explained his surgical plan, the surgeon asked if I wanted to discuss the risks of the operation. I fear I may have laughed and pragmatically said, 'Well, presumably, if you don't do this I am going to die, so the actual numbers are irrelevant.' He smiled, nodded and put the forms in front of me. I quickly added my signature, and as he left the room I felt surprisingly calm. I am an over-thinker, but usually I limit it to things where I feel I can influence the outcome. This was largely outside my control.

8. Relish The Challenge

A jovial anaesthetist came to see me and we had a good chat. My only question was whether he could do anything to stop me being sick as many times as I had been after my last surgery. I was relieved when he said there was good alternative medication, but unfortunately this turned out to be an issue I wished I hadn't raised.

Finally, on the Wednesday afternoon, I escaped my dismal room and was moved to the ward to prepare for surgery. I knew I was going to be first on the surgical list the next day, so there was little to do except sit around and contemplate what was to come. I wasn't scared of dying, and the possibility only occasionally crossed my mind. As in 2005, I was far more concerned about how much of my capabilities I would regain, and if I would be the same person after the operation.

My main fear was a further decline in my physical capacity. I was worried that if, as they suspected, they had to repair my tricuspid valve as well as replace the infected pulmonary, I would end up taking more medication or be further restricted in my capacity for exercise.

What I never doubted was that I was going to survive and come back from this latest challenge just as good as I had been before, if not better. I love the saying 'what doesn't kill you makes you stronger', and I was determined that this would be true. At no point did I question why this was happening to me. I accepted that it was just another part of my journey, and that, far from being a negative, it was supposed to happen exactly as it did.

I am not at all vain or concerned with my appearance, but I wondered how much I would visibly change. My scars have never really bothered me, as they have been a part of my life since childhood. The scar from my first surgery had faded to the faintest of lines by the time of my second operation some twenty-four years later. Then, that had almost disappeared in the intervening twelve years. If you didn't look closely, you probably wouldn't notice. I was occasionally caught completely off guard if someone asked about it.

But here I was, yet again waiting for that same incision to be re-opened. I have always been fortunate in that I seem to heal well. I remember vividly, on one of my trips to the bathroom on the night before surgery, taking off my pyjama top and looking at myself in the mirror. I studied my scar as if to imprint onto my mind how it looked, recognising that no matter what the outcome it would soon be different.

People feel differently about their scars. Some are super-proud of them, seeing them as a badge of honour or a marker of what they have overcome. Others are embarrassed or ashamed, feeling that their scars make them stand out in a negative way. Worse still, they feel disfigured.

I have always been indifferent about my scars, neither hiding them nor going out of my way to have them on display. Displaying a scar is, of course, inescapable when you have a red line from just below your collar bones to the bottom of your ribcage and a selection of lines, dots and divots elsewhere. Most styles of shirt, dress or top show at least the top of it, if not more.

Although the look of my scars doesn't worry me, they do feel odd and I can be quite protective. I had a boyfriend who liked to trace his finger along my sternal scar, something that set off an instant physiological, almost anxious response that I can't easily explain. It is as if the area is more sensitive, and any form of contact triggers unwanted memories.

Early on the morning of my surgery, I was woken up to take my pre-med. I got re-acquainted with the latherless Hibiscrub, which I had to shower in twice, and lay in my freshly changed bed for just a short time before the porters came to take me to theatre. Looking back, I have no recollection of feeling any emotions. It was as if I had detached myself and was more like an observer than an active participant in my life. I assume this is a natural reaction to extreme stress, but I felt totally calm and collected.

I have realised that my ability to separate myself from my feelings during the most stressful situations is a real advantage. I rarely get extremely anxious, as I quickly determine what factors I can and can't control in a situation and focus my energy on those I can. I don't like the feeling of my emotions being out of control – I use logic to separate the raw facts so I can work out more easily if something represents a real or a perceived threat. That level-headedness has proved to be an advantage, and it is only rarely that I find myself experiencing extremes of emotion. If I do, I quickly recognise what is happening and seek to understand why.

The downside to my approach is that it may lead people to think I have it all figured out, as my ability to outwardly express my emotions is held in check. It can feel a bit like being a swan: serene above the surface, but paddling furiously underneath. I have had to learn that there is no shame in sharing my fears, but it is certainly not something that comes naturally.

If I am struggling to deal with a difficult emotion, I try to cover it up with humour. In the anaesthetic room, I can distinctly remember laughing and joking with the doctors and nurses, seemingly oblivious to my precarious situation. Just before he put me to sleep, I can remember relaying to the anaesthetist a quote from one of my favourite movies, *The Second Best Exotic Marigold*

Hotel, in which Sonny says, 'Everything will be all right in the end… so if it is not all right, then it is not yet the end.'

The surgery took four hours, and the first thing I remember was coming round in intensive care. The next few hours were a blur, with various nurses coming and going or simply sitting in my room completing their paperwork. This time I had no recollection of the breathing tube being taken out, but I remember being incredibly uncomfortable, restless and unable to get any respite from the pain. I was connected to a patient-controlled analgesia pump, which allowed me to administer pain medication myself, but no matter how often I pressed the button it didn't seem to make any difference.

At least after my last surgery I was relatively pain-free. This time I was still being sick and I was in agony. I have always been one to accept hardship in life, and I have a high tolerance for pain, but this was a true low point. I clearly remember sobbing to the nurse, 'Please just let me die', as I just didn't know what to do with myself.

It turned out that, rather than the morphine-based pain medication that had made me so sick in 2005, I now had codeine-based drugs. This might have been fine, but to be effective there needs to be a good base level in the blood, so when you press the button it tops up the medication. I was so in and out of it that I couldn't maintain any level at all, so when I pressed the button it didn't seem to have any effect. I reached a point of despair and just resigned myself to it, rationalising that eventually things would improve. There were a lot of conversations in the room about trying unsuccessfully to get my blood pressure down, and doubtless my pain level wasn't helping in that department.

I have never been a fan of pain medication – or, in fact, medication in general. I prefer to work with the idea that if I can take care of my body and help it to stay strong and healthy, I really should be able to look after myself. I do take regular blood thinners, but in hospital I seemed to be rattling with the large number of drugs I had in my body.

My need for control meant that I could never just take any pills or potions I was presented with. Instead, I always examined them to ensure I recognised them and knew why I was taking them. The more astute nurses took the time to point out each of the tablets and give an explanation if I asked. It must be a skill to recognise which patients want to be involved in the nuances of their care and which don't. Some want to know everything, and some don't; there is no right answer and we are all different.

Being in hospital again truly brought home what an onerous and stressful job being a nurse is. One little mistake with a patient's medication can have serious consequences, and with the number of patients each nurse is responsible for, it is remarkable that more issues don't arise. It certainly wouldn't be a good job for someone with my appalling memory!

I have some recollection that one of the surgeon's team came by to explain that the operation had been a success. They had been able to clean up a lot of the infected tissue and replace my pulmonary valve with a new homograft taken from a wonderful person who had opted to donate their organs after death. Having accessed my medical records, I know that the valve came from a 52-year-old woman who had a brain haemorrhage. I can't say thank you, so I will pass on her amazing gesture in kind. The best news was that my tricuspid valve, although leaking badly due to the elevated pressures in my heart, looked undamaged. They left it alone, with the hope that as the size of my heart shrank the valve would stop leaking and return to working well.

Over the next few days, I moved from intensive care to the high dependency ward. My recovery continued to go well, but I had a dramatic reminder of how quickly things could go wrong when the man in the bed beside me had a cardiac arrest late one evening. There may have been a curtain between me and him, but it was still shocking to hear it all happening and to understand how hard the team of doctors and nurses were working to save his life. He ended up having his chest sawn open on the ward so they could keep him alive long enough to get him to theatre. All the while, somebody was on the phone trying desperately to find a surgeon who could get to the hospital in time.

The aftermath didn't make for a restful night of sleep. Although I could rationalise my own fears, it was hard to stop thinking about all that I had heard. I kept replaying the scenario, secretly wondering if the same thing could happen to me. It took me a long time to fall asleep, and I woke the next day to find a new occupant in the bed next to me. I can only hope that the chap somehow survived.

Thankfully, my immediate recovery was much less eventful. I was still massively uncomfortable in my chest and back, my desire to lie still and rest not being satisfied by what I hatefully called my snake bed, which came with me from intensive care. One of the big risks for anyone stuck in bed is pressure sores from lying in one position, so on top of the nurses encouraging me to roll onto my other side every few hours, the bed had a system of inflating tubes, which alternately blew up and let themselves down at regular intervals. It always seemed that just as I was getting some relief, the thing would start moving about beneath me again.

It had also been noted that because I had had a stroke I was at risk of a blood clot, so I had to wear special inflating 'boots' wrapped tightly around my lower legs to prevent the blood pooling in my extremities. If you can imagine lying on the ever-moving snake bed, coupled with this crazy leg-wear, which was operating on a slightly different inflate-to-deflate schedule, then you have some idea of how bizarre and annoying it was. It would have been funny if it wasn't so darned uncomfortable, and I couldn't wait to get out of that bed and away from it. I was rather miffed when the lady opposite me managed to get the nurses to change her special mattress for a normal one – although I asked too, I wasn't so lucky.

I was attached to a large amount of monitoring equipment, and every time I flinched I seemed to set off some alarm or other. My most frequent word was 'sorry', as the poor nurses had to keep coming to my bedside to check on me and reset the equipment. I have a real issue with perceiving myself as a burden, so the hospital environment, where it is hard to do anything for yourself, was hard on me mentally.

Mark drove Mum up for a visit the Sunday after I had left the intensive care unit, as I was keen that she did not come to see me until then. Mum is a remarkably strong woman, but she's much more of a worrier than I am. I wanted to be in a reasonable state before she saw me. Also, if any part of my immediate recovery had been difficult, she wouldn't have been able to do anything other than wait and worry. I have always been grateful that although Dad died at home, Mum wasn't there at the time to feel guilty about what she did or didn't do to save him. The team of paramedics who were in the house when he had his heart attack failed, and I have sought solace in that she had no reason to feel responsible.

I have concluded that it is usually harder for the relatives of someone who is seriously ill than it is for the person themselves. When it is me who is lying in the bed, I at least feel that I have some control over the outcome and what happens to me. For relatives, I can only imagine that it is disempowering and painful to watch someone they love suffering, with little they can do about it. If I could protect my mum from feeling that way, I would. At home, she had friends for support and her familiar routine. I know that they provided some comfort when everything else was so uncertain.

My first attempt to get out of bed and sit in the chair was OK to begin with, but then I started to feel incredibly dizzy and disorientated. The nurses helped me back to bed, assuring me that this was quite normal and just the result of lying down for so long. I was more determined a few hours later and, after an initial wobble, I calmed myself down and managed to spend several hours sitting rather gingerly in the chair. Although everything either hurt or ached, having been in this situation before I knew that if I could just get myself moving, things would rapidly improve.

Over the next few days, slowly but surely the various tubes, drains and wires were removed, and I started to feel a little more human. Once the urinary catheter had been removed and I could move about and get to the bathroom on my own, my next goal was to do whatever I could to be discharged. I knew that I was going back to Derriford, but that would be a big step forward. Some people love the security of being in hospital, but I don't enjoy it at all. In my mind, I had survived the most perilous period, so – fingers crossed – the only way now was back up. I felt more than ready to deal with whatever came next.

Keeping a positive mindset

One of the biggest challenges of living with a long-term health condition can be dealing with uncertainty. We can either be in denial or paralysed by fear, and it is not easy to strike a healthy balance in between. With many of life's obstacles, they arise, we overcome them, and then we move on. Long-term health conditions are more difficult in that they never completely go away. There is a fine line between being aware of what could happen and minimising the risk, as against basing every decision (or making no decision) on a fear of something that is unlikely to happen.

My approach has always been to try and live my life as unfettered by my state of health as I can. There are some inescapable truths about my physical capabilities, which have certainly diminished in recent years, but I can also be overly aware of symptoms or perceive them as more restrictive than they are. I often ask myself whether it is my mind or my body holding me back. At least in asking the question, I must think more deeply and evaluate the truthfulness of my response. I cannot deny my history, but I refuse to let it define me either.

I have also taught myself to focus on what I can still achieve, despite my limitations, rather than berate myself for what I can't. The only failure would be not to do my best with what I have got. It is a continual process of holding on and letting go. We all face the reality of changing expectations as we get older, so I have simply had to adapt to those restrictions a little earlier. On a positive note, there are still so many areas of life in which I can improve, from learning a language to playing an instrument, so the possibilities are endless.

Over the years, I have also come to view my heart condition as my biggest asset and something that positively sets me apart from other people who have not faced similarly significant health challenges. It has taught me many worthwhile lessons about not sweating the small stuff, living in the here and now, compassion and empathy for others, what is truly important to me, and, most of all, a profound sense of gratitude.

I have spoken to many other patients with congenital heart conditions who wish that they hadn't been born with this seeming handicap to face, as they feel it has held them back. I can sympathise with their view, but I truly wouldn't want my life to have played out any differently. I suspect that I would not have pushed myself or achieved what I have if I hadn't faced these challenges.

I suppose it also feels like a waste of energy to imagine myself leading a different life. Whether I choose to embrace it or not, this is my reality, and it is my choice how I interpret it. I can see it purely as a negative or I can use it to my advantage. I strongly believe that I am the person I am because of what has happened to me, and not in spite of it.

CHAPTER 9

Life Doesn't Owe You Anything

*If all misfortunes were laid in one common heap whence
everyone must take an equal portion, most people would be
content to take their own and depart.*

SOCRATES

I was slightly nervous about seeing my chest scar – I feared that it might be an ugly mess, considering that it was my third 'zipper'. I need not have worried. When the long dressing was removed several days after surgery, even the two nurses looked pleasantly surprised. One looked to the other with a smile and said, 'I know who did that!' As I looked down I saw a neat, thin line, with just a few small areas of dried blood.

Much less pleasant, visibly or comfort-wise, has been the scar on my groin. When the surgeon was explaining his pre-operative plan to me as he was getting consent, he said that, as this was going to be my third open-heart surgery, he didn't know what issues he would encounter as he started to access my heart. He wanted to connect me to the cardiopulmonary bypass machine through the femoral artery in my groin before he started cutting away, so, as he phrased it, he had 'got me' before he pushed into the unknown.

Equally, at that point I was very unwell, and I assume many things could have gone wrong before, during or after the operation. The cardiopulmonary bypass (CPB) machine, also known as the heart-lung machine, is designed to supply the body with oxygenated blood and takes on the role of both the heart and lungs during cardiac surgery. An early version of the bypass machine was used during the first successful open-heart surgery in 1952, and it is fascinating to think that before that, little of today's life-saving cardiac surgery was possible. Without its invention, I simply wouldn't be alive!

The other scars I sometimes have to explain are the three 'bullet holes' at the top of my abdomen, just below the bottom of my main scar. They look like three squinting eye sockets, and mark where the chest drains were left after the operation. Anyone who has experienced open-heart surgery will tell you what an 'interesting' experience finally having chest drains removed is. They are somewhat uncomfortable when they are in (they are used to drain any accumulated fluid and blood from the chest cavity after surgery), but it is the strangest sensation to have them unstitched and pulled out of your middle when they are no longer needed.

Add together the three scars down my front, the multiple chest-drain scars from surgeries one, two and three, a scar just above my left breast marking the site of an implanted cardiac monitor, and the new femoral bypass scar, and my body is a map of my journey. My scars are so much a part of me that I am not at all self-conscious about them any more. Sometimes they are a conversation starter, and occasionally I can see people checking them out and not being sure what to say.

I have never hidden my scars or felt ashamed, but I don't go out of my way to have them on show either. I think that has been part of my acceptance process. I am no more or less of a person because of my health history. I have spoken with fellow congenital heart patients who feel upset that we have a mostly hidden illness, which may not be easy for others to recognise. People can be quick to judge, especially if a younger person with no obvious disability parks in a disabled space or causes a hold-up by walking incredibly slowly in a crowded street.

Yet, the flip side is also true. I have spoken with cancer patients who hated having no hair after chemotherapy, as it seemed to label them as a person with cancer who was to be pitied. I also have a friend with an above-the-knee amputation and a prosthetic leg, who gets fed up with people who don't know him thinking that he needs help with everything. I suspect that, like me, his disability has driven him to be fiercely independent and to achieve more in life than he might have done otherwise.

The reality is that we all have our issues in life, be they physical, mental, emotional, financial or otherwise. The only way to treat someone else is with honesty and respect, doing our best to learn about them and their lives through first-hand conversation. We shouldn't judge them or make assumptions, which so often turn out to be incorrect. Never judge a book by its cover!

Late in the afternoon on Monday 10 April I was moved onto a ward, in a gloriously big room with three other ladies. Vastly different from the dismal coronary care unit downstairs where I had started my journey, it had an enormous row of windows looking out of the back of the building onto a little strip of woodland. When the blinds were closed every night, I made sure to leave a little strip at the end next to my bed, and several times I saw a handsome dog fox walking precariously along on the high wall. I could see bluebells and spring flowers, and with the windows slightly open, listen to the sound of birdsong. I might not have been allowed to leave the ward, but there were reminders everywhere of how good it was to be alive.

Just as I had done after my previous surgery all those years ago, I started my regular exercise routine. It might have only counted as little more than a shuffle, but I desperately needed to feel that I was being proactive in my recovery. As I started to feel more like myself, I began to pass the time by striking up conversation with the other people I found prowling the corridor. One of these was a lovely lady who was a keen cyclist and, like me, keen to get back into her previous activities.

I am not at all gregarious and I favour my own company, but it felt pretty good to allay someone's fears about their recovery using the amount of experience I had to draw on. Most of the people I spoke to were getting over their first surgery, often for acquired rather than congenital heart disease, so I had every sympathy for the huge shock their new circumstances had given them.

I have often noted how blessed I feel to have known about my issues all my life. Although unexpected issues have arisen at surprising times, I have always known rationally that there would be challenges ahead. I know from speaking with my clients who have had health issues hit them out of the blue, often later in life, how hard that period of adjustment can be.

On the Thursday evening, just a week after my surgery, I was transferred the 120 miles back to Derriford to continue my treatment and antibiotic regime. The journey back was a lot less eventful than the delivery trip, but unfortunately it took place in what could well have been the world's most uncomfortable ambulance. It was best suited to short trips delivering nearby patients to their hospital appointments, and not motorway driving. Being bounced around for hours left me in absolute agony. This situation wasn't helped when, because nobody at Derriford seemed to be expecting me, neither my pain medication nor my long-overdue antibiotics could be sorted out until gone 2am. It was another low point, when I was left sobbing in the bed, completely unable to sleep.

The next day I moved wards again, this time to the room where I would spend much of my time for the next five and a half weeks. Getting back to Plymouth was a positive step. Not only was it much easier for my mum, friends and clients to visit, but I was back on familiar ground. I had realised from early on in this episode that getting upset about my situation wasn't going to help, and I was ready to make the most of the opportunity.

The only very difficult time in Derriford came just a few days later. After I had been free to wander the hospital and had started to build a new routine, infection control got wind of my return from Bristol and put me in quarantine while they tested me for a new superbug. It would have been bad enough with the regulation five days of isolation in my room, everyone having to 'glove and gown' whenever they entered, but due to some 'procedural difficulties' involving the use of the wrong swabs, my stay was extended to eight days.

I am afraid that I didn't handle it well. Having made so much effort to get myself up and moving about while I was in Bristol, this captivity seemed like a giant step backward. My frustration wasn't helped by the obvious fact that if I was harbouring this bug, I was likely to have already spread it to people on several wards, the restaurant, the coffee shop and the Macmillan Centre over the preceding four days!

I dealt with the initial confinement stoically, but as the days drew out and nobody seemed entirely sure what was going on, I am ashamed to say I became grumpy and, ultimately, cross. Although I knew rationally that nobody was deliberately out to make my life difficult and that it was the process rather than people who were at fault, I let my emotions get the better of me. On day eight, I declared in no uncertain terms that unless somebody took responsibility for sorting out my situation, I was going to make a formal complaint. Unsurprisingly, I was released and free to get back to my wandering just a few hours later!

Looking back, I have sought to understand why I found my confinement so difficult. I wasn't just slightly bothered by the situation, but incredibly anxious and upset. My deep-seated beliefs and sense of control were being challenged, so I lost my objectivity and ability to assess the situation, and instead defaulted to a learned behaviour.

The staff on the ward were excellent. I was in the privileged position of being probably the least needy patient. Providing I got my intravenous antibiotics four times a day and took my other medication, I didn't need much help. I did my best to minimise the time the nurses and domestic staff needed to spend in my room, and in return I appreciated the autonomy I had. At one point, I was given permission to catch a bus from the hospital into the city centre to have lunch with Paul, a congenital heart friend from Liverpool who was attending a business meeting.

My friend, Fiona, even drove me to my cottage so I could do a quick bit of paperwork (mainly paying bills) and find a few items that my mum had been unable to locate. Several times each week, I managed to walk out of the hospital grounds to the gym where I have been a member for much of the last thirteen years, to share breakfast with my friends. Those little glimpses of normal life helped me to stay optimistic and positive and were a real boost to my spirits. They certainly allowed me to be less unsettled by the other, not so normal aspects of my situation.

Another fortuitous thing that happened a few days after my return from Bristol was that the consultant cardiologist who had been overseeing my care since my previous consultant retired, came to see me. He was excellent in trying to get to the bottom of why I had my stroke, and here again, after my endocarditis, he did a thorough review. On looking at my drug chart, he immediately suggested that since my infection markers were continuing to fall, I should be taken off the gentamicin, a particularly aggressive antibiotic with side effects of damage to the inner ear, balance and hearing.

That attentiveness to detail probably saved me from a wobbly life where I would have been unable to ride my bike, surf or do the activities I enjoy. Thankfully, the only lasting effect from the amount of the drug I had already been given seems to be mild tinnitus. Amusingly, when I had been out of hospital for many weeks, I was about to accuse my neighbour of running a dehumidifier all night. It took a while to realise that the drone was coming from my own ears and not next door!

I have often pondered the relationship between a doctor and a patient with a lifelong illness; it is not like the interactions between a doctor and patient who only know each other for a short while. Congenital heart disease is never fully cured, and a lifetime of follow-up is usually required. As an educated patient with a good understanding of my condition, I have always appreciated that the specialist consultants who have overseen my care throughout my life, have been prepared to work with me in all aspects of managing my condition.

The congenital heart specialist nurses in Bristol and Plymouth have also had an incredibly positive impact on my care. As the contact point between me and my doctors, they have the unenviable task of translating my rare, but generally significant, needs into a relevant appointment or referral. Their reassuring smiles and calmness have been particularly welcome during my various hospital inpatient stays, when I can find myself feeling very alone and out of control. The challenges of being a lifelong congenital heart patient have undoubtedly been made easier by the amazing medical professionals in my life.

I try hard not to seek medical help unless I really think I need it, and this has not helped my situation at times. The most obvious examples are the twelve years I spent without any follow-up, and the many weeks I wandered around with endocarditis, desperately unwell but foolishly believing that I had everything under control. I can be my own worst enemy!

That makes me wonder what factors determine how well people cope when facing a life-changing medical diagnosis. Some shun all but essential medical support and have few concerns, yet others become dependent and reach out for advice on every possible symptom. The stress on NHS services means that all too often the resources are only in place to deal with immediate medical concerns, and there are fewer resources to help with the psychological impact of living with a long-term health condition.

It is widely known that cancer patients, who often have a long and arduous treatment journey, can feel incredibly alone when they no longer have that regular interaction with nursing and medical staff. They can be essentially left to get on with their life and deal with the psychological impact of what has happened with little or no support. Charities like Macmillan recognise this void and can support people through that transition, but not everyone knows how to reach out for that help or even wants to. NHS psychological support for people with long-term illnesses is not routinely offered, so it can be hard to access. This leaves many people vulnerable and suffering more than they should.

I have always been pragmatic about the challenges I have faced. Much of that has come down to being proactive about understanding my condition and working hard to overcome its limitations, while at the same time accepting that I can't fix everything. Life doesn't come with a coping manual for stressful situations. What one person finds easy to deal with may knock another completely off track. I believe that resilience is a learned skill, and one that can be nurtured.

One of the recognised assets for anyone dealing with trauma is the ability to find benefits. Rather than dwelling on what you have lost, the idea is to look for what you have gained. I did this a lot while I was in hospital, and it undoubtedly made the experience more bearable. When else in life was I going to have this much time without any real responsibility? I didn't have to cook, clean, do the laundry, go to work, make the bed or anything else I had to do in my normal life. My only obligations were to be in my room four times a day for antibiotic infusions, blood tests and ward rounds.

Some people might think the freedom to sit all day, watch TV, sleep and relax would be a blessing, but I found it quite disconcerting. I felt reasonably well and not like I needed to be stuck in hospital, but the antibiotics couldn't be administered any other way. As someone who thrives on routine, I knew that the only way I was going to look after my mental health was to set myself tasks that would keep my mind busy.

I created a daily exercise routine, building up from being able to leave the ward and make it as far as the main entrance, to being able to circle the main building, to reaching the coffee shop at the edge of the site. The goal was to get out at least three times a day, between breakfast and lunch, lunch and dinner, and dinner and bedtime. Weather permitting, that is what happened.

The biggest boon was discovering that there was a nature reserve just behind the hospital, with easy access from the rear car park. There were mapped walks of varying lengths, frequent places to sit and rest, trees to shelter me from the spring showers and plenty of wildlife to amuse and occupy me. Most days, at least one of my walks included the reserve. I only made one judgement error, when a wrong turn meant that what I thought would be a twenty-minute walk took nearer to fifty-five – and, more worryingly, I didn't see another soul. I started to imagine a scenario with police helicopters looking for a missing patient!

I also needed an intellectual focus to keep me occupied, so I enrolled in several online courses on mindfulness, life coaching, psychology, grammar and punctuation. I was determined not to waste any of this gifted time, and I hoped to leave the hospital having moved towards several of my life goals – one of which was writing this book.

Keeping busy gave me a real sense of retaining control. All too often when we encounter big obstacles in life, we stop our normal habits, give up exercising, eat less healthy food and withdraw from social situations. That can leave us vulnerable to a negative spiral of self-loathing and depression. I knew that I needed to be proactive in looking after my mental and physical health, and be aware of any less healthy protective patterns that were creeping in.

I kept up as many of my normal habits as I could: I got up and went to bed at my regular times, ate the same breakfast, got out of my pyjamas and into my comfortable clothes and took daily exercise. That routine gave me a sense of stability and normality, allowing the rest of my brain adequate space to cope with the less controllable aspects of my situation. Although I wouldn't say that I enjoyed my time in hospital, I coped with it far better than I expected to.

I was careful not to look back with regret or to wonder if different choices could have changed the outcome, as that would have been pointless. Instead I tried to look forward, and I proactively spent time planning and defining my future. I knew that the long hours I had been working had been draining my limited energy levels and making me less willing to engage in other areas of my life.

I assessed my priorities and reluctantly decided to stop the fitness aspect of my work. I was sad to lose clients I enjoyed working with, many of whom had been with me for years, but I knew that if I was to sustain my business I had to be more respectful of my capabilities. Leaving the house at 6am and returning thirteen hours later was no longer an option.

While I have known chemotherapy patients use the same PICC line for many months, mine got blocked at least once a week. Each time, a special solution had to be used to dissolve the clots, and invariably I missed one of my antibiotic infusions while it was sorted. The easy solution was to insert a temporary cannula, but I had a miraculous ability to knock it out and decorate the room with blood, usually during one of my nightly visits to the bathroom. More than once I had to press the emergency button and then watch in shame as a poor nurse had to mop the floor to clean up the blood.

Another area where I struggled psychologically while in hospital was in always being receptive to the requests from my friends and clients who wanted to come and visit. I am a true introvert, and at times I felt rather trapped by the stream of visitors coming in to what was, in effect, my new home. In normal circumstances I would have been able to balance my social interaction with my need for quiet 'me time', but in hospital it wasn't so easy to protect my personal space.

I was already at the mercy of the doctors and nurses, and I felt conflicted by reconciling my need for privacy with what I perceived as the expectations of others, who, after all, only meant well. Not a day passed when I didn't have at least one visitor, and sometimes it was as many as three or four. I knew I should feel grateful that people were making the effort, and most of the time I did appreciate it, but in an email to a friend I likened my situation to being an animal in a zoo. I struggled greatly with being seen when vulnerable or not at my best, and, looking back, I realise how much anxiety it caused me.

Things came to a head when, recognising that I was in a dire financial position with no income and enormous monthly outgoings, one group of clients started a crowdfunding campaign and another began collecting donations. I didn't know how to react appropriately, and it made me feel hugely and irrationally upset. I had an overwhelming sense of guilt, which I couldn't dismiss. I know that I did not handle myself well or, indeed, know how to accurately express what was bothering me without causing further offence. For that, I am sorry.

I was quite taken aback by how humiliated and upset I felt. The feelings were so strong that it was very hard for me to understand them or express why I was finding it so upsetting. It was not until I spent time afterwards analysing my feelings that I could get to the bottom of the real issue. Looking back, I recognised that my emotions were triggered by a challenge to several of my core beliefs. This is a good reminder that if we find ourselves over-reacting or being unreasonable in what should be a simple situation, there are likely to be some deeper issues at play.

Core beliefs

We do not randomly make decisions. Instead, we base our thoughts and hence our actions on a set of beliefs, many of which start to form in childhood. We formulate beliefs about ourselves, other people, the world around us and the future. Our minds filter every thought to decide how it fits in with our beliefs, and this then influences how we think and act.

Many of our core beliefs are beneficial in our lives, but others can lead us to make unhelpful assumptions. Negative core beliefs can leave us feeling inferior, unlovable, destined to be unhappy, or that bad things are bound to happen.

Speaking to hundreds of people with long-term medical conditions has shown me that our core beliefs can be challenged in many areas.

If you believe that your value in society is based around your job, how does that stand up if you become unwell and unable to work? How do you then preserve your self-esteem?

If you are strongly independent and think asking for help shows weakness, how will you see yourself if you must rely heavily on others? Will you feel guilty or inferior?

If you believe that it is unfair to expect someone to love you because of your illness, what are your chances of forming a meaningful relationship? Are you more likely to push people away?

If you believe that the world is completely fair and you get what you deserve, what happens when you receive a life-changing diagnosis? Are you automatically a bad person?

If you believe it is only a matter of time before you have another setback, how do you plan your future with optimism? Will you lead less of a life because of that 'what if' fear?

As you read through those questions, you might think to yourself 'I never feel like that'. That is what I thought as well, until I purposefully spent time looking at my core beliefs and I saw how they had affected so many of my life choices and actions. I can admit that at different times and to varying degrees, my thoughts have been directly affected by every one of the beliefs represented by those questions.

The power comes when you recognise that you are feeling them, analyse what has triggered that reaction, and decide if this is going to help or hinder your progress. Whereas we can all recognise that some situations make us feel a certain way, it can be harder to identify our core beliefs. I find it easiest to ask 'what' questions so I can dig deeper into my thought processes:

- What would happen if this thought were true?
- What is so bad about that?
- What would that say or mean about me or my situation?

'What' questions force us to analyse what our beliefs mean, rather than just looking at why we feel a certain way. Asking why we feel the way we do is likely to lead to us justifying our response or being defensive.

If I look at my own situation – feeling so uncomfortable about people wanting to help me – I could ask the following questions:

What are you feeling?
Upset, irritated, verging on angry.

What is making you feel that way?
I am not a charity case.

What would be so bad about that?
Other people deserve it more than I do. I don't want to feel like a burden.

Ironically, I know that part of experiencing gratitude is to be willing to receive as much as to want to give – evidently, I still have some work to do. Is it that I don't feel worthy when people care? Do I deserve to be loved? Does showing my vulnerability make me less of a person?

This inner conflict reminds me that although I have come far in understanding my sense of self, who I am and what I stand for, I still have much to learn.

CHAPTER 10

You Only Live Once

Gratitude radiates out from me in all directions, touching everything in my world, and returns to me as more to be grateful for. The more gratitude I feel, the more I am aware that the supply is endless.

LOUISE HAY

I hope that my story is far from over. I often joke that having survived this far, despite the grim reaper's many attempts to take me, I must still have unfinished business to complete.

I am rebuilding myself and bouncing back yet again, using all the skills and lessons I have learned along the way. I am not sure if it has got any easier, as I am still having to put in the physical and mental work, but perhaps with a clearer map of the process I at least know what to expect.

I am notoriously impatient, and I find it hard not to feel down about the fitness I have lost, the opportunities I have missed and the inevitable difficulties on the road ahead. If I could wave a magic wand and have everything go back to normal, I would. I must remind myself that part of the growth process after any big life event is to take the time to assimilate our new identity and come to terms with the changes we have been forced to make. The process can't be rushed or forced, or issues will be left unresolved and come back to haunt us later.

It seems appropriate to share some of the key areas I am focussing on to be proactive in aiding my recovery. My advice is not comprehensive, and it is only proven in so much as it has worked for me. It is not intended to replace the guidance of a medical professional, but if you find yourself facing a medical trauma – or, indeed, any big life trauma – I hope it will help.

Supporting your recovery

Eat well

I love the simplicity of the idea that we are what we eat. In their rawest form, the nutrients and energy we get from our food are the power our cells need to give us energy to move, repair and rejuvenate. Emotional or physical trauma demands more energy. Think of the quantity and quality of your nutrition as the fuel in your petrol tank. Add dirty, low-quality fuel and your car isn't going to run efficiently and it will, at some point, break down.

I am a big believer in focussing on the quality of the food we put into our bodies, as by doing so the quantity and nutritional profile take care of themselves. Whatever your dietary preferences, it makes sense to eat unprocessed food most of the time, because this is usually lower in unwanted calories, additives, preservatives and chemicals. Plus, by cooking our own food from raw ingredients, we have a much better understanding of what we are eating, and more appreciation about where it comes from.

We often lose appetite when we are unwell, just when our body is craving extra calories to assist in healing. Meals you have prepared and put in the freezer can be a boon, as can simple choices like soups and stews. Losing a lot of weight while you're unwell can slow down your recovery, so try to find food that you enjoy and is easy to eat.

Of course, this is never easy if you are in hospital and at the whim of the menu, which always sounds way better than it tastes! Within a few weeks of my most recent hospitalisation, I got to the point where I couldn't bear to eat another baked potato. Once I was mobile enough, I was desperate to access a wider variety of foods of my choosing. Thankfully there was an M&S Food store in the foyer, and they sold a great selection of pre-prepared salads and healthy meals. With a lack of accessible cooking facilities, I became quite adept at persuading the nurses to microwave things for me, and I saw more than a few jealous looks from other patients as I took my dish back to my room.

Similarly, rather than the inevitable crisps and chocolate, I encouraged visitors to bring me fruit, vegetables and nuts. Occasional treats were fine, but I was aware that I was significantly less active than normal, so I was wary about overindulging. Doing the best I could with the resources I had was the key.

Exercise

It would be hard for me, as an exercise professional, not to touch on the power of exercise to promote healing and recovery. Our bodies are designed to move, and, according to a 2011 Department of Health report, 'regular physical activity can reduce the risk of many chronic conditions, including heart disease, stroke, Type 2 diabetes, cancer, obesity, mental health problems and musculoskeletal conditions.' Regular exercise not only promotes our physical health, but it helps with the mental side as well.

It can be hard to think about exercise when you're facing a potentially life-changing situation, but being active is a simple way to take back control and establish a routine. It is a misconception that to be good for us, exercise must be intense, sweaty and unpleasant – something as simple as a gentle walk in nature can have countless benefits for the mind and body. Set a goal, make a plan, start small, monitor your progress and adjust your plan as necessary.

If you don't come from a fitness background, it can be hard to make a start. We all know that exercise is good for us, but living with a health condition often throws more obstacles in our way. We can only start from where we are today and determine to be better. If anyone with your health condition has ever achieved something, then you have the potential to work towards it as well. You may never get there, but you will still be better than you are today!

I am a firm believer in exercising with others when possible. It is much easier to be consistent about exercising if we have some company. I always appreciated it when my hospital visitors accompanied me on my daily rambles, even if it was only as far as the coffee shop.

Even when I was confined to my room (or worse still, the bed), I still did my best to move what parts of my body I could as often as possible. I always feel better when I am able to move around regularly. When you are already sore and cranky, sitting around seems to compound the discomfort. I am a fan of getting outside into the fresh air if you can, as it can be such a boost to the spirits.

Physical activity has become my therapy. It is a commitment to myself to do my bit to stay as fit and strong as possible. The deck may not be stacked in my favour, but that is all the more reason to do my part and not allow poor health choices to add to my problems. If I use my health as an excuse, I am only letting myself down.

Stick to a routine

It is easy to get out of our routine when we are facing a crisis. Often, having our independence stripped away robs us of the activities, social interaction and sense of purpose we normally feel. If you are stuck in hospital, it can be hard to do anything other than accept the imposed routine, but it is possible to build around it.

On my most recent hospitalisation, I made a schedule for eating, personal hygiene, studying, exercising, e-mailing and so on. It also included some free time. I believe that sticking to that routine saved my mental health. Aside from being surprisingly productive, I was never bored or at a loss for something to do.

Actively scheduling regular times for eating, sleeping, exercising and social time can help to bring order and normality to a day when so many other things are uncertain. Focussing on the things I could control prevented me from dwelling on the rest.

Keep a positive mindset

Throughout this book, you will find details of how I have dealt with the medical challenges that have come my way. If you are facing your own medical adversity, my advice is to spend regular time working through your feelings, understanding your reactions and taking control of your emotions.

Given my history, it is perhaps unsurprising that I have occasionally suffered with poor mental health. Luckily, it hasn't been for extended periods and I have always been able to pull myself up. I am sure that my levels of self-awareness have helped. I have learned to take full responsibility for everything that has happened in my life – not as a way of chastising myself, but to avoid shifting power to something or someone else.

If I default to the mindset that I am responsible, that also means that I have the opportunity to do something about it. It can be hard when it feels like everything is against me, but sitting in the corner snivelling about it won't change the outcome. I strongly believe that we make our own luck, and life is easier if we are optimistic. If you acknowledge that your emotions are completely under your control, then you have the power to feel however you want to.

If I recognise that I am going down a negative pathway, the first thing I do is acknowledge my feelings. It is no use denying them or trying to supress those thoughts. Often, I deliberately indulge them, but I allow myself a strict five-minute time frame for this, after which I must move on. Hal Elrod, bestselling author of *The Miracle Morning* (2017), calls this the five-minute rule, and practising this has transformed my ability to deal with my emotions more effectively.

I also like the idea that we can smother negative emotions by distracting the mind and forcing it to focus on a positive activity. Positive and negative emotions cannot exist at the same time. It may sound silly, but laughing, singing, jumping up and down or pulling faces in the mirror can flip that switch and prevent the anxiety and rumination that often accompany negative thoughts.

Life is simply much more pleasant when we choose to live in a positive mindset. There may well be future challenges to face and unexpected difficulties to overcome, but I believe that everything is going to be OK. That doesn't mean looking at life through rose-tinted spectacles or living in denial, but recognising that you have the option to view everything in a positive light.

Best of all, positivity brings like-minded people into your life. My own resilience has been boosted since I surrounded myself with friends who share a similar view and have the courage to call me out when I am not living up to my own values. That attitude also repels people who will actively drag me down or drain my reserves. I used to think that being locked in self-pity would draw compassionate people towards me, but in fact it did the opposite. We all like to assist people who want to help themselves and will make the first move, not those who look to everyone but themselves for answers. It's not all about us!

Practise mindfulness and meditation

This topic can be quite deep, so if you want to develop your own daily practice then I would advise you to seek out some help on the subject. Personally, I enjoy using some of the guided meditation apps such as Headspace, Calm or Buddhify, as they have allowed me to figure out which formats work best for me. In my younger years, I was resistant to the idea of spirituality and self-awareness, yet as I have got older I have gained an appreciation for how important it is to our health and wellbeing.

Facing any form of medical trauma or diagnosis can leave us feeling disconnected, both from ourselves and from the world around us. That uncertainty builds anxiety, which can push us further off track and away from who we want to be. When our current reality is uncomfortable, it is easy to dwell on the past or our fears for the future, rather than focussing on the factors we can control in the here and now.

It has taken me many years to stick with regular meditation and mindfulness, and even now I let life get in the way all too often.

What I have experienced is the increased calm and self-awareness that has come with daily practice, so I would strongly advise you to give it a try. I find some of the online apps helpful, as they give me a regular reminder of the importance of consistency, but you need to decide what works best for you.

Keep a journal

I kept a diary every day until I was in my late teens, but it wasn't until a few years ago that I took up the habit again. These days, it is less of a blow by blow account of my day than a setting of my expectations, goals and progress.

I try to write in my diary twice a day, although often it happens only once. My morning ritual is to write down three things I am grateful for, three goals I would like to accomplish and three emotions I would like to feel that day. My evening review looks at how I fared, sometimes giving more detail about any adversity, learning or outcomes.

Keeping a journal is perhaps the most powerful way I have gained a better understanding of myself and what makes me tick. Even though it might not always make for comfortable reading, looking back can act as a powerful reminder of the progress you are making and how far you have come.

I also love having a clear focus for what I want to achieve each day. If you follow my technique, you don't have to set big goals – the act of ticking off the simple stuff, like getting a haircut or walking to the shops, can give you a much-needed sense of achievement. It is all relative to your state of mind and ambition at the time.

Try expressive writing

This follows on rather neatly from the suggestion above. It's something I have been doing for much of my life, without realising that there was a name for it. Many challenges bring change, and we are forced to look in detail at who we were before, how we have evolved and where we are going. That takes time, and processing all the information is not always easy.

I have always found that writing down my thoughts and feelings makes me feel more powerful, and in doing so I have achieved a level of acceptance that I might not otherwise have done. Something about the act of putting things down on paper clears my head and enables me to be more objective about what I am thinking.

More recently, I learned about the work of Dr James Pennebaker at the University of Texas. He researched how expressive writing could help people to deal with emotional challenges. He found that for expressive writing to be effective, we need to detail not only the facts of our situation but also our emotions and thoughts, reflecting on how we feel.

I often write letters to myself as a way of working through my thoughts. Sometimes I keep my reflections, and sometimes I don't. It doesn't have to be pretty – spelling and punctuation don't matter. It isn't meant to be shared, as this would make us feel the need to censor ourselves, and in doing so be less open or honest.

Pennebaker found that people who spent fifteen minutes a day, on four consecutive days, following his advice, experienced mental and physical health benefits. His studies have also shown that expressive writing can help to improve your mood, control symptoms, lower blood pressure, reduce visits to the doctor and even boost memory. For me, expressive writing has enabled me to make sense of my experiences and resolve conflict that could have a negative effect on my life.

Build a support network

I have always been lucky to have the wonderful support of close family and friends as I journey through my medical mystery tour. Many studies, such as those mentioned in the book *Upside* by Jim Rendon, detail how having the support of close friends and family can be an important asset in helping recovery. It can boost your immune system, reduce depression, and improve mental and physical wellbeing.

I know first-hand that it is easy to feel isolated and depressed when facing a potentially life-changing illness. As I have noted before, my instinct leads me to push people away and withdraw when I feel vulnerable – not the best reaction to support my mental health. My levels of self-awareness allow me to recognise what is happening, though, and put safeguards in place to help myself.

A social support structure is important for anyone facing a medical trauma. We all need that close friend or family member to confide in, to share our worries and fears, and to shoulder some of the psychological burden. A shared experience in a time of stress can massively strengthen a relationship.

From a practical point of view, if I end up in hospital, having people I can rely on to water the plants at home, bring me clean clothes and keep an eye on things gives me more time to focus on getting well. I have always been lucky that my friends, knowing how much I dislike hospital food, make it their mission to bring me as much fresh fruit, vegetables and healthy snacks as possible.

We need to pick our supporters carefully, as not everyone is well suited to this role. Sometimes, family members can be too close to the emotional situation. It is no good if your previously level-headed and reliable friend can't cope with you being the centre of attention for a while or feels threatened when your view of yourself and your identity changes.

Find the right people, and a support network is an absolute boon. I honestly don't know how I would have coped with almost two months in hospital without the support of Mum, Mark, Rachel, Chris and Paul. Just having that friendly voice on the phone or a short visit was often all I needed to transform an otherwise difficult day. I will be forever grateful.

Find (or build) a community that shares your story

It is easy to believe that you are alone in facing your particular adversity. Yet there are people who, even if their stories do not mirror yours, share experiences. It is natural in a crisis for friends and family to rally round, but they drift away as they get back to their normal lives once the immediate crisis has passed. We can experience loneliness or isolation when this happens, so it is important to reach out to others for help.

If you have a long-term illness, the physical scars may fade but the mental ones can take longer to heal. There is nothing quite like talking at length with another human being who truly understands your fears, shares your emotions and empathises with your experiences. It can also inspire us that it is still possible to have a meaningful life after a diagnosis.

Post-traumatic growth doesn't just happen for individual people, but can take place in a group when everyone is focused on the same outcome. For me, the most power comes from a group that promotes ways to move on, rather than dwells on the adversity itself. What makes Race for Life in the UK and Team in Training in the USA so successful is that they not only raise awareness of a health issue but often provide athletic goals for patients themselves.

In the Invictus Games, all participants come from a service background. These people have faced a multitude of challenges, which have dramatically changed the course of their lives, and they have come back together in the spirit of defining a new narrative for their story. It is not just about their physical and mental injuries, but about celebrating the people they have become.

Virtual groups can also offer a huge amount of emotional support. In the online world, I can connect with fellow congenital heart patients from around the world, giving me a setting to share my struggles and victories with people who can truly understand how I feel. Perhaps, most of all, I feel less alone knowing that I have a community of friends who share many aspects of my story.

Of course, some people naturally eschew support groups, as they act as an ongoing reminder of experiences they would rather forget. In my own experience, it has been most helpful to dip in and out of support groups based on my needs at the time. For a healthy balance, I also keep up regular social activities and relationships outside that environment.

Reconnect with your sense of purpose

I was introduced to the concept of finding my 'ikigai' by Pete Cohen, founder of the Mi365 life coaching community. 'Ikigai' is a Japanese word that means 'a reason for living', or, in more Western terms, having a life purpose.

When we are immersed in a health challenge, it is easy to become so focused on the day-to-day issues that we forget there is a life beyond the current situation. Even when the future seems bleak, if we lose the ability to stay upbeat then hope is lost.

I was probably in my thirties before I had a clear vision of who I was and the legacy I wanted to leave. That coincided with a developing awareness that I couldn't take my future for granted and that every day was another step closer to my end. Rather than being a morbid thought, that motivated me to ensure that my life counted for something – that if I did it right, my influence would continue after I had gone.

For many people, that legacy involves their children, but for a variety of reasons that is not the case for me. Over the years, my individual goals may have changed and become more focused on others, but my overall mission has remained much the same. It should come as no surprise that my legacy is to inspire anyone facing a medical adversity to see beyond their limitations, to believe in themselves and to nurture their passion so they can lead an amazing life.

I have coached people over the years who can't clearly define their life purpose. This was often because they were over-thinking it or expected it to be an enormous revelation. If you don't know what your life purpose is, this is an opportunity to give it some thought. What makes you happy? What activities do you enjoy? If you didn't have to work for a living, what would you do? What would your ideal day look like? What will people say about you after your death?

Of course, it can be hard to integrate our life purpose completely with the need to make a living, but I tend to find the closer we get, then the happier we become. Over the years, I have been very fortunate to love my work, and if I ever started to resent it or find it less appealing, then I have made a change. The constant reminder that life is short has perhaps made me more aware than many of the need to enjoy as many moments as possible, and not to sacrifice my long-term happiness for short-term financial gain.

As shown by so many of the observations in this book, learning about ourselves and what makes us tick can be an uncomfortable process. One of my overriding life goals is not to find myself on my deathbed filled with regret. Every day is an opportunity to get closer to leading my dream life, at peace with my life choices, with who I am and what I am, and fulfilling my ikigai. I want nothing more than the same for you.

Giving back

I believe that when we feel able to move beyond focussing on ourselves to start improving the lives of others, that is the catalyst for true post-traumatic growth. At times, dealing with my health problems feels as overwhelming as being up to my eyeballs, in the swamp, with the alligators. It is only when I have worked through my emotions, feel in control of most aspects of my life and can see a clear future path, that I am again able to give back. For me, this is the ultimate goal of recovery.

How we choose to give back is, of course, a personal decision. Some people choose to link a physical or mental goal with charity fundraising, others join or set up a support group where they can share their experiences for the good of others, and yet more work on awareness-raising activities. It doesn't matter how you do it, as long as you have a genuine desire to help others.

I never used to be comfortable with sharing my story, for fear that it would have a negative effect on how other people saw me. I am long since over that illusion – I know that the people who matter will judge me kindly.

There is a power in sharing our story, whether this is with large audiences or just one person. We never know when our openness and willingness to share will make a real difference to somebody else's life. Writing this book has certainly been therapeutic for me, but I hope more than anything that its legacy is to inspire courage and optimism in you.

Conclusion

Reading back through these ten chapters makes me realise how far I have come. From that shy child, to the depressed young adult, to a now self-aware middle-aged woman. The big medical challenges I have faced have undoubtedly shaped my character and made me who I am. If there was an opportunity to change any of it, I honestly wouldn't.

My mental resilience and optimism have been nurtured over many years of having to face up to my mortality, the uncertainty that comes with living with a long-term health condition, and the desire to keep pushing my boundaries.

My ability to understand and control my emotions has been the biggest differentiator in my life. Once I learned to take absolute responsibility for who I am, and that I always have a choice in how I react to the things that happen to me, my challenges became much easier to cope with.

I don't believe that I am in any way unusual in my approach. My upbeat attitude was born out of necessity and the recognition that I didn't like the alternative. I haven't always followed a smooth learning curve and there have been moments where I have had serious wobbles and let myself down, yet this is not a life of regret.

I have let go of anger, sadness and guilt, and in its place the main thing I feel is gratitude. I am unbelievably lucky to live where I do, to have access to life-saving medical services and to receive the unwavering support of my friends and family.

I know that I am getting closer to living up to my life's purpose. My mission to help others thrive in the face of medical adversity is imprinted on my soul and motivates so much of what I do. Sadly, I don't have children, so instead my legacy is in the positive difference I can make in the lives of others while I am here.

Rather like Doug, who so changed the course of my life when I was at university, I believe that every interaction is a chance to pass on that gift. I hope that, like the ripples in a pond, my impact expands beyond those in my immediate circle. It's a lofty goal, and one that I am always working towards.

It acts as a constant reminder to always show the best version of me that I can, to treat everyone with love and respect, and to be generous in giving my time and energy to support others. Ironically, far from detracting from my ability to lead a fulfilling life, I have discovered that those positive moments always come back tenfold!

Our health is perhaps our most precious commodity, yet it is perhaps the least valued until it is in jeopardy. We are all likely to be affected by major health challenges at some point, and they strike at the core of everything we think about ourselves and the world around us.

Staying upbeat

Whenever those hardships come, and in whatever form, I hope that by reading my story you feel better equipped to deal with them. For me, finding ways to stay upbeat in the face of life-changing diagnoses has not prevented those challenges, but it has certainly made them easier to live with.

I would love to hear from you and to learn more about your story. Contact me at

Twitter: @Bethfit
Facebook: www.facebook.com/BethJGreenaway
Website: www.MerlinFitness.com

References

Campbell, J. (2008), *The Hero with a Thousand Faces: The Collected Works of Joseph Campbell*, 3rd edition. Novato, CA: New World Library.

Cohen, P. Mi365 online coaching community. Available at www.Mi365.me.

Department of Health (2011), *Start Active, Stay Active: A Report on Physical Activity for Health from the Four Home Countries' Chief Medical Officers*.

Elrod, H. (2017), *The Miracle Morning: The Not So Obvious Secret Which Will Transform Your Life Before 8am*. London: John Murray Learning.

Frankl, V. E. (1984) *Man's Search for Meaning*. New York: Simon and Schuster.

Joseph, S. (2012), *What Doesn't Kill Us: A Guide to Overcoming Adversity and Moving Forward*. London: Piatkus.

Kubler-Ross, E. (2008), *On Death and Dying: What the Dying Have to Teach Doctors, Nurses, Clergy and Their Own Families*. London: Routledge.

Pennebaker, J. W. (2004), *Writing To Heal: A Guided Journal for Recovering from Trauma and Emotional Upheaval.* Oakland, CA: New Harbinger.

Pennebaker, J. W. (1997), *Opening Up: The Healing Power of Expressing Emotions.* New York: Academic Press.

Rendon, J. (2015), *Upside: The New Science of Post Traumatic Growth.* New York: Touchstone.

Seligman, M. E. P. (1999), The President's Address, *American Psychologist,* 54, pp. 559–562.

Seligman, M. E. P. (2006), *Learned Optimism: How to Change Your Mind and Your Life.* New York: Vintage Books.

Snyder, C. R. (1994), *The Psychology of Hope.* New York: Free Press.

Tedeschi, R. G. and Calhoun, L. G. (1996), The Posttraumatic Growth Inventory: Measuring the Positive Legacy of Trauma, *Journal of Traumatic Stress,* 9, pp. 455–471.

Mindfulness and meditation apps

Headspace (www.headspace.com),
Buddhify (www.buddhify.com),
Calm (www.calm.com)

Acknowledgements

This book is dedicated to my friends and family, who have not only supported me through my darkest hours but joined me in celebrating my many victories. Without them, my bumpy journey would have been a lot less fun.

A huge thank you must also go to the many teams of medical professionals who have kept my heart beating over the years. Their care and compassion has allowed me to lead an incredibly fulfilling life, not defined by my health or history.

Lastly, but by no means least, my amazing mum and late father, who brought me up to see beyond my limitations and to make the most of every opportunity. My sense of gratitude knows no bounds.

The Author

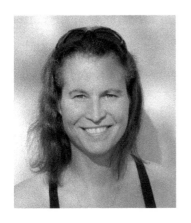

Beth Greenaway is living proof that we do not need to live a life defined by the adversities we have had to face. Born with serious congenital heart defects, she has always been incredibly grateful for the medical intervention that has enabled her to survive. Keen to make the most of every day, she has led a varied career, working as everything from a small business computer engineer to a farm livestock inspector.

In spite of her variable health, which has continued to throw obstacles in her path, she has always tried to follow an active lifestyle. While living in the USA in her 20s and early 30s, she qualified as a personal trainer and enjoyed living the life of a competitive recreational triathlete, racing everything up to Ironman distance. Her dedication to putting in the necessary hours of training allowed her to compensate for her lack of physical ability.

In 2012, her passion for helping anyone to experience the joy of exercise, particularly those with long-term health conditions, led her to open a rehab studio in Plymouth, where she now runs a variety of specialist classes. Her ethos is very much to celebrate what we can still achieve, rather than to dwell on what we can't. Always one to find the positives in any situation, her mission is to inspire people to push their own limits and to never give in.

Having overcome a stroke in 2016 and then a life-threatening endocarditis infection just a year later, which resulted in her third open-heart surgery, she feels well positioned to help others facing similar struggles. Never one to allow her health to hold her back, she still loves training in the gym, riding her bike, and splashing about in a variety of water sports.

She lives in a little blue and white cottage in the Cornish countryside, surrounded by bicycles, kayaks, surfboards, boats and associated kit. Hobbies requiring less equipment may have been more practical!

Twitter: @Bethfit
Facebook: www.facebook.com/BethJGreenaway
Website: www.MerlinFitness.com

Lightning Source UK Ltd.
Milton Keynes UK
UKHW02f0309010618
323562UK00007B/442/P